Practice Management for the Medical Office

POWERED BY

SimChart® for the medical office

D1307089

Practice Management for the Medical Office

POWERED BY

SimChart® for the medical office

ELSEVIER

ELSEVIER

3251 Riverport Lane
St. Louis, Missouri 63043

PRACTICE MANAGEMENT FOR THE MEDICAL OFFICE
POWERED BY SIMCHART FOR THE MEDICAL OFFICE   ISBN: 978-0-323-43012-8

Notices

Knowledge and best practice in this field are constantly changing. As new research and experience broaden our understanding, changes in research methods, professional practices, or medical treatment may become necessary.

Practitioners and researchers must always rely on their own experience and knowledge in evaluating and using any information, methods, compounds, or experiments described herein. In using such information or methods they should be mindful of their own safety and the safety of others, including parties for whom they have a professional responsibility.

With respect to any drug or pharmaceutical products identified, readers are advised to check the most current information provided (i) on procedures featured or (ii) by the manufacturer of each product to be administered, to verify the recommended dose or formula, the method and duration of administration, and contraindications. It is the responsibility of practitioners, relying on their own experience and knowledge of their patients, to make diagnoses, to determine dosages and the best treatment for each individual patient, and to take all appropriate safety precautions.

To the fullest extent of the law, neither the Publisher nor the authors, contributors, or editors, assume any liability for any injury and/or damage to persons or property as a matter of products liability, negligence or otherwise, or from any use or operation of any methods, products, instructions, or ideas contained in the material herein.

Library of Congress Cataloging-in-Publication Data

Title: Practice management for the medical office powered by SimChart for the
    medical office.
Description: St. Louis, Missouri : Elsevier, [2016]
Identifiers: LCCN 2015036376 | ISBN 9780323430128
Subjects: LCSH: Medicine--Data processing. | Medical
    offices--Management--Data processing.
Classification: LCC R858 .P72 2016 | DDC 610.285--dc23 LC record available at http://lccn.loc.gov/2015036376

Content Strategist: Jennifer Janson
Content Development Manager: Luke Held
Content Development Specialist: Heather Rippetoe
Publishing Services Manager: Jeff Patterson
Project Manager: Lisa A. P. Bushey
Designer: Ashley Miner

Printed in the United States of America

Last digit is the print number: 9 8 7 6 5 4 3 2 1

Reviewers

Starra Robinson Herring
Director
Medical Assisting Program
Stanly Community College
Albermarle, North Carolina

Jeanne E. Lawo, RN, MSN
Clinical Site Manager
SLUCare at University Tower
St. Louis, Missouri

Julie Pepper, CMA, (AAMA)
Instructor
Medical Assisting Program
Chippewa Valley Technical College
Eau Claire, Wisconsin

Preface

Practice Management for the Medical Office Powered by SimChart for the Medical Office was developed to provide step-by-step guidance in using the practice management features of SimChart for the Medical Office, with a strong focus on the functions of the back office. With all of the helpful materials provided within the program, this text will walk you and your students through the medical office workflow, providing practice with completing superbills, submitting claims, and reporting functionality and other forms and processes necessary for running a medical practice.

Additionally, three new providers have been added to the Walden Martin Family Medical Group:
1. David Kahn, MD, a dermatologist, which allows for more specific skin treatments with the possibility for some outpatient procedures and testing that might not have been typical to a general practitioner.
2. Angela Perez, MD, a gastroenterologist, also allowing for expanded procedures and diagnoses, as well as inpatient and outpatient procedures.
3. Patrick Taylor, DDS, a dentist, which opens up an entirely new set of procedures and claims opportunities for students. NOTE: Unlike the medical procedure codes in SimChart for the Medical Office, the dental codes do **not** reflect codes that exist in the medical community. These were generated for practice purposes only.

Organization

The text is organized into six units:
1. **Navigating SimChart for the Medical Office.** This unit introduces the student to the product and provides background on the three modules, the simulation playground and EHR Exercises, the encoder, and some of the typical workflow steps surrounding practice management.
2. **Scheduling Appointments and Patient Registration.** This unit introduces students to the calendar and tasks specific to getting new patients registered and scheduling appointments for new and existing patients.
3. **Claim Entry.** This unit introduces students to the superbill, or encounter form, and the process of submitting claims for patient encounters.
4. **Payment Posting.** This unit introduces students to the Patient Ledger and when and how different payments and charges are documented to it.
5. **Reports.** This unit introduces students to the many different forms and reports used to keep the office running and profitable. Students will explore the Day Sheet, the Bank Deposit Slip, and the various different reporting features and functionality within the Coding & Billing module of SimChart for the Medical Office.
6. **Comprehensive Cases.** This unit provides individual case studies that allows students to put together all that they've learned throughout the text. They will walk through four individual cases of new patients that need same-day appointments at Walden-Martin Family Medical Group. They will complete the superbill and submit claims for each encounter and will then be asked to complete some of the final reporting that is typical to a medical practice.

Quick Tips

The following are some tips that will help you to use SimChart for the Medical Office to the fullest.

Familiarize Yourself with Instructor Resources. Access Instructor Resources as often as needed; whenever you have a question regarding a process or where to locate a particular feature. Watch *A Guided Tour of SimChart for the Medical Office* before logging in to SimChart for the Medical Office for the first time.

Use the Student Review Questions on the Evolve site. Although these questions on Evolve are available for student self-study, they can be assigned for a grade that will automatically feed to the gradebook.

To the Student

Practice Management for the Medical Office Powered by SimChart for the Medical Office will provide you with unique, hands-on learning of the simulated medical office. The assignments in this text provide realistic practice of the tasks you will encounter in a real medical office—from front office (administrative) skills to practice management skills (billing, coding, and insurance).

Earning a degree for any role within a medical practice is a rigorous undertaking. The student must gain a complete understanding of how a medical office functions, from the time the patient makes an appointment until the insurance carrier pays for the services provided in the encounter and beyond. Following are tips on becoming a successful student in your field.

Quick Tips

Familiarize Yourself With Student Resources. Review all of the resource materials before class and refer to them whenever you have a question regarding a particular process or feature in SimChart for the Medical Office.

Follow Your Instructor's Lead. Instructors can incorporate SimChart for the Medical Office into the classroom in several ways. Follow instructions regarding how and when to use the application.

Access the Simulation. There are two methods of accessing SimChart for the Medical Office:

- The **Simulation Playground** is the practice environment where you can log in to practice different skills in preparation for completing assignments in the text. You have the option of clearing all of the work completed in this environment of SimChart for the Medical Office.
- The **EHR Exercises** environment is where you will complete the assignments for this text. Your instructor will be able to view your work, and you will not have the option of clearing your work with each new session.

Save Your Work. Almost every screen has a **Save** button. Be sure to save your work in all screens before progressing or exiting. You can even save work within an assignment before submitting, making it easy to return and continue.

Use Available Resources. Instructors are the best resource, but they can't answer questions if students don't ask them. If one student has a question, another student probably does too, so you will be doing everyone a favor by asking.

- Ask your instructor questions after class or during office hours if you are uncomfortable asking during class.
- Email your instructor if questions arise outside of class.

Fellow students are another great resource. Social networking sites can also be a great way to stay in contact outside of class.

- Form study groups to review content on an ongoing basis or to prepare for exams.
- Create a Facebook group for a specific class and post questions and/or study tools for everyone to access.

Textbooks are the basis for most class content. Glossaries, indexes, and online resources can provide additional details about unfamiliar terms and topics.

- List questions from the chapter before class and ask the instructor if your questions are not answered during class.
- Make notes and highlight important content.

Teamwork. The ability to work well with others is an invaluable tool in the workforce. Group projects are a great opportunity to develop interpersonal skills that will make you an asset to any team.

- Volunteer to be the leader of the group or use your people skills to bring out the quiet one in the group.
- If you are typically the quiet member of a group, offer at least one suggestion during every group meeting.
- Practice active listening and do not interrupt. Avoid distractions. Give the person you are speaking with your undivided attention so you process the message.
- Body language can sometimes convey more than words. Observing the body language of others while you are delivering a message will help you to determine if they are receiving the intended message.
- Respect diversity. Understanding that people come from different backgrounds will facilitate collaboration. Team players are respectful of everyone's opinion.

- Gossiping is destructive to a productive learning and work environment. The impact of gossiping can hurt feelings and induce anger, neither of which help to create a positive environment.

Be Considerate. Group projects can also serve as an opportunity to develop skills that help you cooperate with all types of personalities. Remember that practicing consideration will not go unnoticed. Your instructor will remember the example you set, which will come in handy when you ask them to provide a referral letter.

- Be considerate of all classmates in and out of class.
- Do not interrupt your teacher or your classmates because this is rude and disruptive.
- Remember that everyone comes from different backgrounds, so keep an open mind and learn from what others share in class.
- Do not gossip. Gossip damages relationships and is unprofessional.

Be Professional. Approaching school as if it were a job allows you to start developing your professionalism skills the moment you start your medical assistant program. Consistent attendance helps you retain more information, participating in class demonstrates that you are engaged in class discussion, balancing priorities helps you to be prepared for any unexpected scheduling complications, and adhering to established policies will help you succeed.

- Participate in class. You do not have to raise your hand to answer every question, but you should always be engaged in class discussion.
- Determine daycare details in advance and establish a backup plan in case your transportation falls through.
- Keep a calendar to track all of your commitments and be realistic about how long activities really take.
- Contact your instructor immediately if absence is unavoidable.
- Follow the dress code. If you are not already required to follow a dress code while in school, you will certainly have a dress code for practicum.
- Make sure scrubs are in good condition. Pants should not drag on the floor, and tops should be an appropriate length.
- Cover tattoos and remove visible body piercings.
- Always behave professionally when dressed in scrubs and avoid going out socially in scrubs because it could reflect poorly upon healthcare professions.

Work Ethic. Taking responsibility for your education and seeking clarification when you don't understand something in class will help you develop the habit of ensuring comprehension in the workplace. This will ultimately help you to provide the best patient care possible.

- Do your own work and credit your sources. Understand plagiarism and its consequences. Allowing others to use your work is still considered cheating.
- Complete all assignments before the due date and remember that you receive the grade you earn; instructors do not "give" grades.
- Always clean up after yourself. Whether you are in the lab or in a lecture, make sure that your workspace is as clean as or cleaner than when you sat down.

Job Readiness Skills. Many of the skills needed to obtain and maintain a job can be developed while a student is still in a Medical Assistant program.

Positive Mental Attitude. Nobody wants to work with someone who always has a negative outlook. Those who tend to see the worst should use this time as an opportunity to start changing their mindset.

- Keep your self-talk positive. When presented with a difficult situation, identify an aspect of the situation that will benefit the patient, organization, or staff.
- Smile, even when you don't feel like it. Smiling can help create positive interactions, which contribute to a positive environment overall.
- Embrace change. Change is inevitable, especially in health care. Viewing change as an opportunity to learn and improve rather than a chore can also contribute to a positive environment. Try to identify how change can benefit the patient, organization, and staff.

Time Management. Time management is a skill needed for school, as well as work. Figuring out how to balance priorities while in school can carry over to your work.

- Determine daycare details in advance. Having a plan in place when your child or daycare provider is sick can help to minimize schedule complications. Investigate the options available in your area. Is there a center that accepts sick children? Can a close friend or family member care for your child?

- Secure reliable transportation or establish a backup plan if you have car trouble. Know the bus routes and ask other students or coworkers about carpooling.
- Keep a calendar to track all of your commitments and prevent double-booking. Most cellular phones provide a calendar function and paper agendas are also available. Whichever version you prefer, keep it current with your work schedule, personal activities, and family activities.
- Be realistic about how long activities really take. For example, if you don't have more than 1 hour available for a dentist appointment and you know that traffic is always hectic, you should choose another day for the appointment.

Lifelong Learning. Change occurs frequently in health care, and developing tools to help with staying current in your field will make you a better medical assistant.

- Join your national and local professional organization.
- The American Association of Medical Assistants (CMA [AAMA]) provides continuing education opportunities including an annual national convention, *CMA Today* magazine, membership in the state organization that provides opportunities at a more local level, and online and paper-based CEUs.
- The American Medical Technologists (RMA) provides an annual national meeting, AMT State Society meetings, and online and paper-based CEUs.
- Find workshops and seminars that promote new skill development or update existing skills. For example, diagnostic and procedural coding manuals are updated every year. Attending a workshop regarding this topic will ensure that you are using current coding criteria. Requesting information and demonstrations from manufacturers when they release laboratory tests or equipment is another good way to remain current.

Dressing for Success. Because health care is a conservative field, follow the dress code policy at all times.

- Cover tattoos and remove visible body piercings. Some dress code policies even go so far as to state that there can only be one earring in each ear.
- If scrubs are required, make sure they are in good condition. Pants should not drag on the floor, and tops should be an appropriate length.
- Some positions require business casual attire. If unsure as to what clothes are allowed, be sure to ask. Business casual is not the same as casual clothing worn at home. Sweatpants, yoga pants, shorts, midriff-baring tops, flip-flops, shirts with logos or statements, and halter tops are not appropriate.

Resume Building. All of the skills obtained in school help to build a resume that will attract potential employers. Welcome every opportunity to learn a new skill, and showcase these skills in your resume.

- Create a portfolio with examples of different skills learned, such as a business letter written using Microsoft Word, a project organized using Microsoft Excel, samples of EHR documentation using an application such as SimChart for the Medical Office, and a checklist of clinical and administrative skills gained during practicum. Refer to Appendix A for more information.
- List experience using software programs such as SimChart for the Medical Office, Microsoft Word, Microsoft Excel, Microsoft PowerPoint, or Microsoft Access. Include extracurricular activities such as tutoring or involvement in any student or professional organizations. This type of background demonstrates a willingness to expand beyond the basics required in school.

Contents

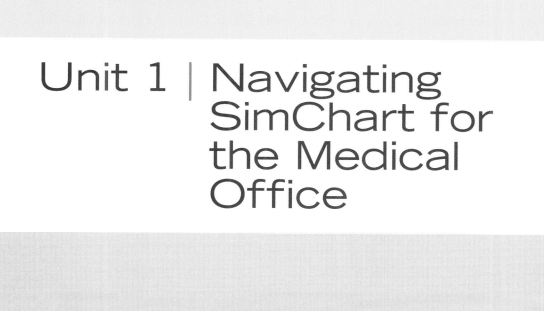

Unit 1 | Navigating SimChart for the Medical Office

About SimChart for the Medical Office

SimChart for the Medical Office is a comprehensive practice management and electronic health record (EHR) system that includes both the administrative and clinical functionality of a medical practice. You are able to experience the flow of data in a simulated setting, seeing the entire workflow from scheduling appointments, registering a patient, and charting in an electronic record to posting charges and payments, performing coding and billing services, and auditing for compliance all within one product.

There are three methods of accessing the functionality of SimChart for the Medical Office: the Simulation Playground, the EHR Exercises, and via the prebuilt assignments within the product itself. For the purposes of this text, we will discuss the first two.

Simulation Playground

The Simulation Playground is the practice environment of SimChart for the Medical Office (Figure 1-1). Although the same functionality is available in assignments, the Simulation Playground gives students an opportunity to familiarize themselves with simulation features before completing any assignments. Students can review an assignment description and practice the assignment in the Simulation Playground before beginning the graded assignment. This practice can help students become familiar with identifying the steps necessary to complete an assignment. Upon reentering the Simulation Playground, students can choose to continue work or clear previous work to begin a new session (Figure 1-2). Additionally, instructors can use this environment to create their own assignments.

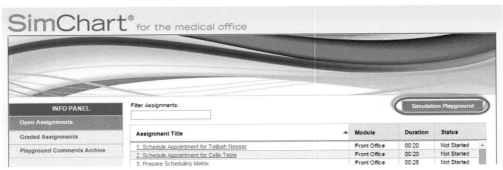

Figure 1-1 Access to the Simulation Playground.

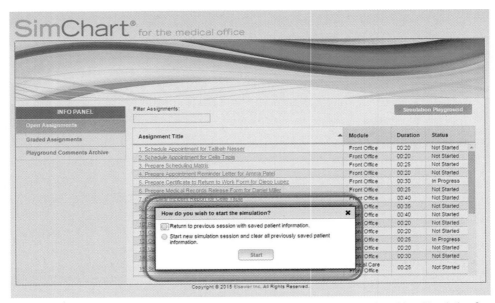

Figure 1-2 Simulation Playground Radio Buttons: Return to Previous Session or Start New Simulation Session.

EHR Exercises

The EHR Exercises part of SimChart for the Medical Office (Figure 1-3) has all of the same features and functionality as the Simulation Playground, but does not give students the option of starting fresh with each login. This serves the dual purpose of preventing the accidental deletion of text assignments and facilitating support and grading by instructors. Because of this functionality, all assignments in this text will be performed in the EHR Exercises.

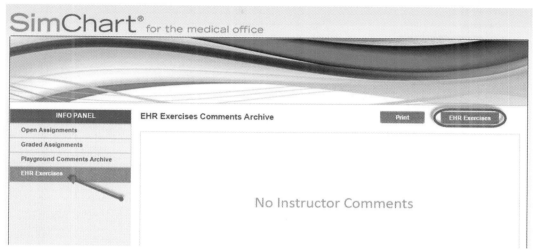

Figure 1-3 EHR Exercises Button.

Modules

SimChart for the Medical Office is organized within three modules, which contain the main aspects of the medical office workflow: Front Office, Clinical Care, and Coding & Billing (Figure 1-4). The default landing page upon entering the simulation is the Front Office Calendar to represent opening the medical office for the day. From that point, users can navigate freely throughout all of the modules of the medical office workflow in order to practice or accomplish the specific tasks of an assignment.

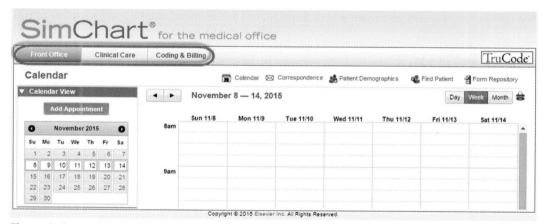

Figure 1-4 The Three Modules of SimChart for the Medical Office: Front Office, Clinical Care, and Coding & Billing.

Front Office

The Front Office Module of SimChart for the Medical Office contains the calendar and the functionality of scheduling appointments and other tasks specific to the front office. The calendar shows all appointments for the week unless a filter is selected. The calendar can be filtered by Provider, Appointment Type, or Exam Room (Figure 1-5). Filtering by Provider shows only the patient appointments specific to one provider at Walden-Martin Family Medical Clinic. Filtering by Appointment Type limits the view to specific types of patient appointments or blocked time for providers. Filtering by Exam Room allows you to see all appointments that have been scheduled to a specific room.

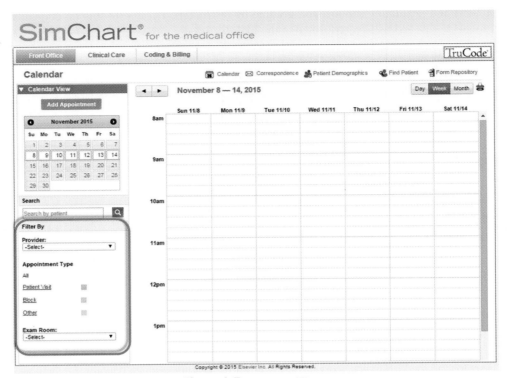

Figure 1-5 Calendar Filters.

In addition to filtering the calendar, it is also possible to change the view. The bottom left corner of the screen has two buttons for viewing the calendar: Exam Room View and Provider View. Exam Room View gives a daily look at the appointments scheduled in each room (Figure 1-6). Note that if exam rooms are not assigned when scheduling patient appointments, nothing will populate in this

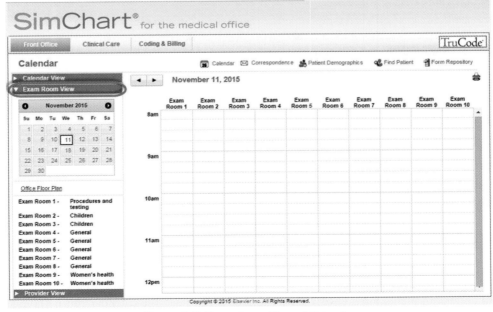

Figure 1-6 Exam Room View of Calendar.

calendar. It is also in this view of the calendar that you will have access to the Office Floor Plan of Walden-Martin Family Medical Practice (Figure 1-7). Selecting Provider View at the bottom left of the screen will give a daily look at each provider's schedule.

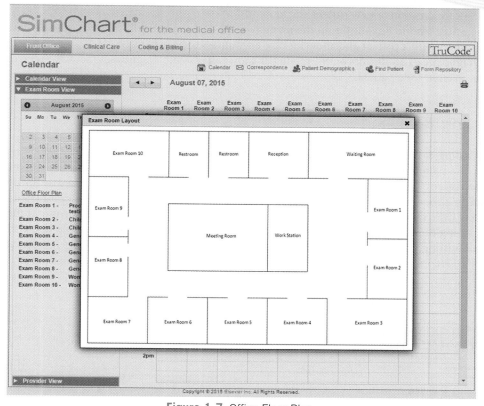

Figure 1-7 Office Floor Plan.

Clinical Care

The Clinical Care module of SimChart for the Medical Office is where the patient charting is completed. Essentially any documentation that needs to be associated with a specific patient is done in this module.

To use the clinical care module in SimChart for the Medical Office, you must select a patient. With a patient selected, an **Info Panel** will appear on the left of the screen providing a menu bar of different options for charting (Figure 1-8).

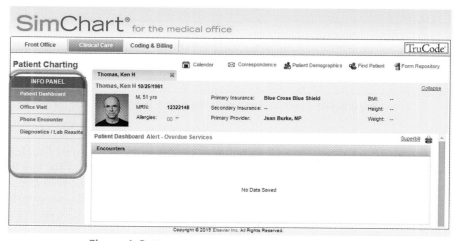

Figure 1-8 The Info Panel in the Clinical Care Module.

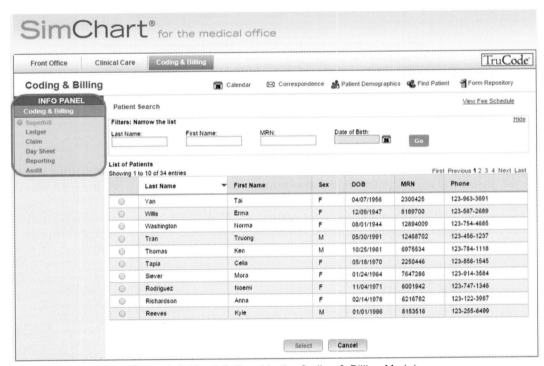

- The **Patient Dashboard** is an overview of encounters, contact information, and other items specific to the patient's plan of care. The bottom of the dashboard contains any forms that have been provided to or by the patient.
- Selecting **Office Visit** on the menu bar will show all existing encounters a patient may have and allow for creation of new patient encounters.
- Selecting **Phone Encounter** on the menu bar, like Office Visit, will show all existing phone encounters with a patient and allow for new encounters to be generated.
- **Diagnostics/Lab Results** on the menu bar shows all labs and diagnostics that have been ordered or received for a patient.

Coding & Billing

The Coding & Billing Module is where a patient encounter is completed and any reporting takes place. If a patient or insurance company makes a payment on a patient account it is documented in the patient **Ledger** and the practice's **Day Sheet**, both of which are accessed from the **Info Panel** in this module (Figure 1-9). Additionally, encounters that have been completed in the Clinical Care module can now be used to generate **Superbills**, also known as encounter forms, in the Coding & Billing module. After superbills have been completed, this module will also allow for submitting **Claims**. Claims can be processed electronically using SimChart for the Medical Office's 5010 compliant documentation or exported into a populated paper claim output.

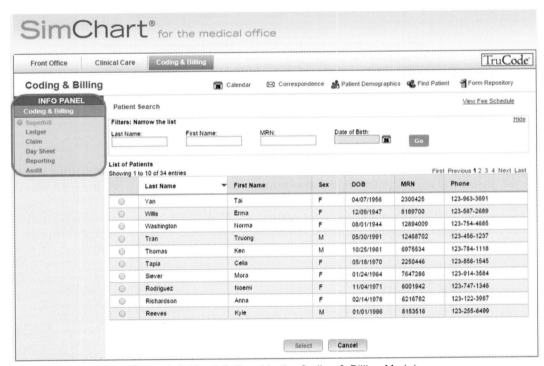

Figure 1-9 The Info Panel in the Coding & Billing Module.

Because superbills and claims are used for billing of procedures, it is also in this module that the Fee Schedule can be accessed (Figure 1-10). This document is a listing of all of the fees for each of the encounters and procedures for Walden-Martin Family Medical Clinic, and is an important tool for completing the superbill and claim process in the Coding & Billing module (see Appendix A).

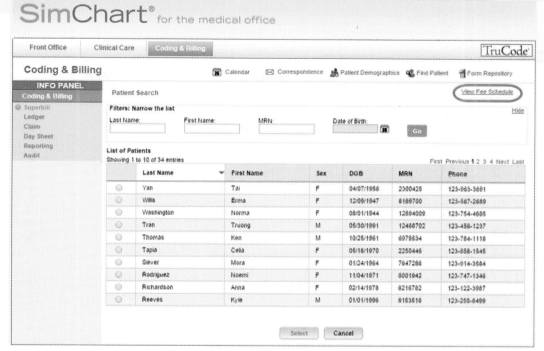

Figure 1-10 Fee Schedule.

In addition to completing tasks specific to patient encounters, the Coding & Billing module of SimChart for the Medical Office offers another important feature for any efficient medical office: **Reporting**. Two different reporting features are offered in this software:

- **Usage** (by either procedure or diagnosis) – This functionality allows for generating reports of patients who were seen in the practice for specific procedures or with specific conditions.
- **Aging** (by either patient or insurance) – This functionality allows for generating reports on outstanding balances categorized by the number of days past due.

Encoder

The TruCode encoder tool is an electronic medical coding resource to use when documenting diagnoses or procedures in SimChart for the Medical Office. This tool can be used to refine and populate codes into encounters, superbills, and claims. Since SimChart for the Medical Office is intended for educational use, a limited set of CPT codes is available within the tool. There are two ways to access the encoder:

1. Clicking the TruCode button in the top right corner opens the tool in a new tab to use as reference while navigating throughout the application. This button is always visible throughout the application (Figure 1-11).
2. Placing a cursor in a field that requires coding will reveal an additional TruCode button. Accessing the tool this way will autopopulate the selected code where the cursor is placed in the simulation (Figure 1-12).

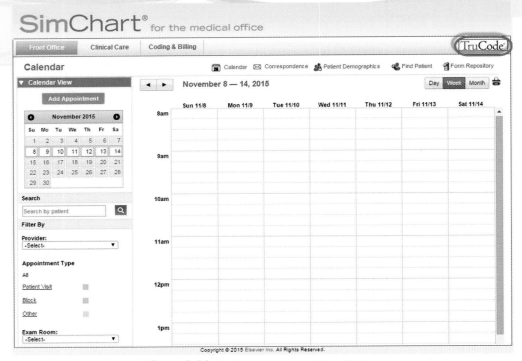

Figure 1-11 TruCode encoder via the Button.

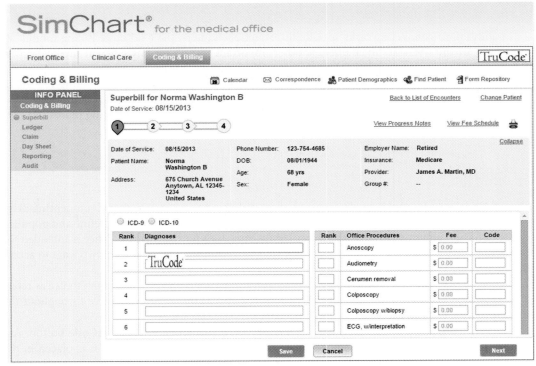

Figure 1-12 TruCode encoder via an Active Field.

Performing a Search

Use the search field at the top of the screen to search for codes by terms or code (Figure 1-13). The following code manuals are included:

- **ICD-10-CM Diagnosis and External Cause** – These books consist of an alphabetic index where you can look up terms and a tabular of codes, which includes all instructional notes.
- **ICD-10-PCS Procedure** – This book consists of an alphabetic index where you can look up terms and a table where you choose the specifics of the procedure to construct the ICD-10-PCS procedure code.

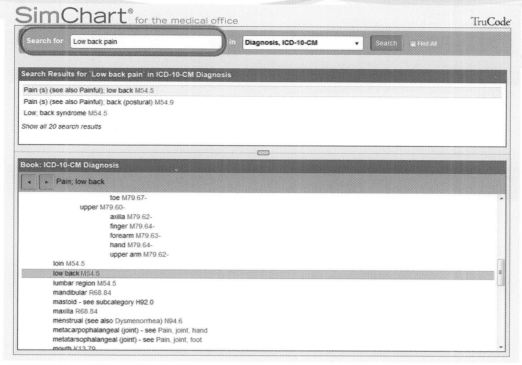

Figure 1-13 Searching by Code Type.

- **ICD-9-CM Diagnosis**, **E Code**, and **Procedure** – These books consist of an alphabetic index where you can look up terms and a tabular of codes, including all instructional notes.
- **CPT** and **HCPCS** – In these books, both the index and tabular are searched simultaneously and tabular results are displayed based on the search.

NOTE: Dental codes are not available via the encoder. Please use the Fee Schedule to look up the simulated dental codes.

Search Results

The alphabetic index appears in the search results when a code book is searched by terms (except for CPT and HCPCS). The Search Results pane displays all index entries from the alphabetic index that match the search terms (Figure 1-14).

If a code has an instructional note, the symbol ▣ appears to the left of the code when the code is highlighted. Instructional notes contain Includes, Excludes, and Notes from the chapter, section, and category levels.

- To view the note, click the symbol (Figure 1-15).

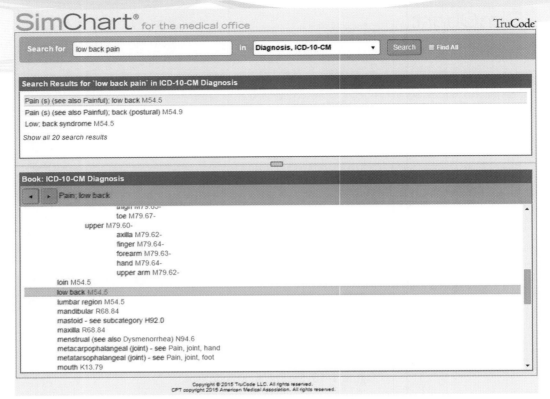

Figure 1-14 The Search Results Pane.

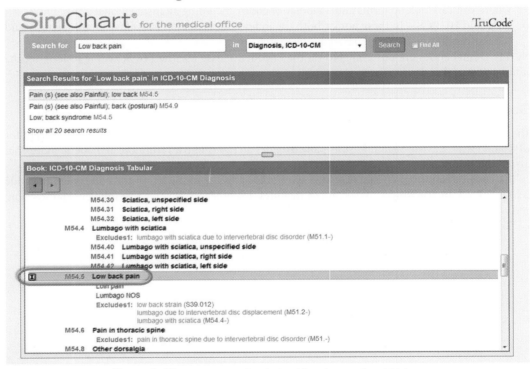

Figure 1-15 Clicking the Symbol to View Instructional Notes.

Documentation

Documentation options vary depending on access point.

- Accessing the Encoder tool by clicking the TruCode button in the top right corner opens the tool in a new tab to use as reference while navigating throughout the application. In order to document this way, copy the desired code and paste it into the correct field within the simulation.

- Accessing the Encoder tool by placing a cursor in a field requiring coding reveals an additional TruCode button and will autopopulate the selected code where the cursor is placed in the simulation (Figure 1-16).
- Expand the list of codes beneath the desired code by clicking the code associated with a diagnosis (Figure 1-17).

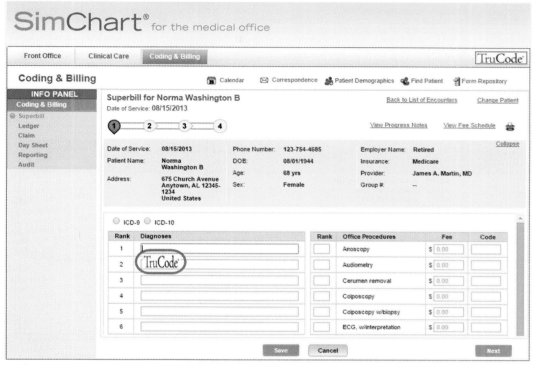

Figure 1-16 Autopopulating the Code by Placing the Cursor in the Desired Area of the Simulation.

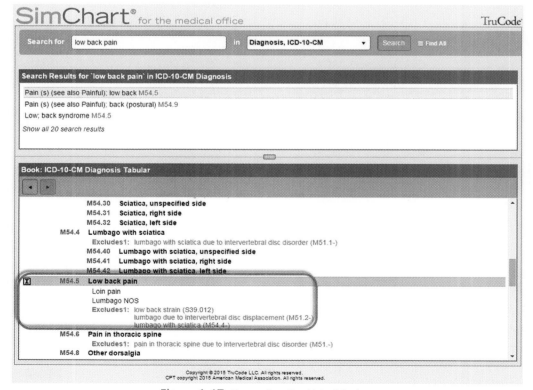

Figure 1-17 Expanding the List of Codes.

- After expanding a diagnosis to confirm that it is the most specific code available, click the code that appears in red in order to autopopulate it within the simulation and continue documenting (Figures 1-18 and 1-19).

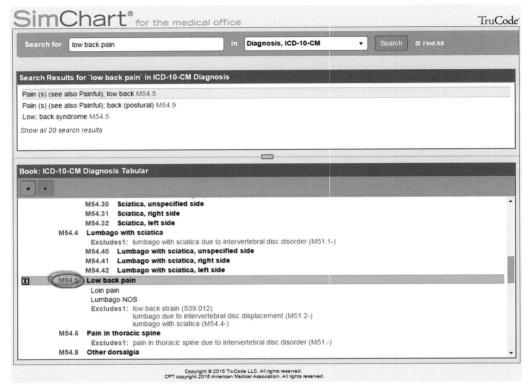

Figure 1-18 Click on the Code That Appears in Red.

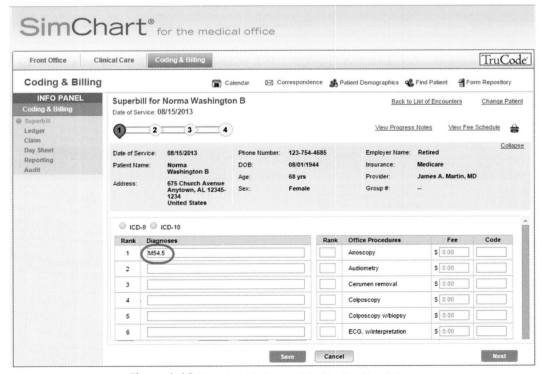

Figure 1-19 The Code Autopopulated in the Simulation.

Common Icons

At the top of SimChart for the Medical Office are common icons that are not specific to any of the three modules (Figure 1-20).

- Selecting the **Calendar** icon will take you to the calendar view of the front office. Here you can schedule appointments by selecting the Add Appointment button or clicking within the actual calendar.
- Selecting the **Correspondence** icon displays the email, letter, and phone communication templates available for use in the medical office. Once a method of correspondence is selected, you will have to complete a patient search in order to assign that correspondence to the patient.
- Selecting the **Patient Demographics** icon will open a search function for you to look up demographic information on an existing patient or add a new patient. It is always important to double check that a patient doesn't already exist in the system before adding.
- Selecting the **Find Patient** icon takes you to the Clinical Care module, where you can search for existing patients. Once you select a patient, his or her record will open for you to review any existing encounters and add new ones.
- Selecting the **Form Repository** icon displays patient and office form templates to use in the medical office (Figure 1-21). Performing a patient search after selecting a form unlocks a form for editing and saves any changes to that patient's record.

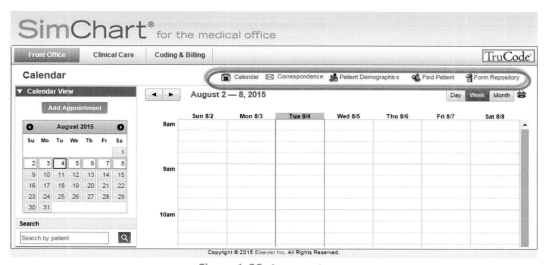

Figure 1-20 Common Icons.

Practice Management Workflow Tasks

SimChart for the Medical Office provides a realistic environment in which to practice common tasks encountered in medical offices, such as scheduling appointments, registering new patients, posting payments, coding, billing, and running activity and aging reports. Walden-Martin Family Medical Clinic includes generalist and specialist providers, which allows students to experience a wide variety of scheduling and billing situations. The following units will provide a sampling of each to ensure a truly comprehensive experience.

In the next unit (Unit 2) you will gain experience scheduling appointments and registering new patients in the system. Ensuring that these two tasks are done correctly and thoroughly will not only keep a practice running smoothly, but also will reduce the risks of claims being denied later in the cycle of a patient visit.

Unit 3 covers the important task of completing a patient superbill in the system and submitting a claim. The superbill documents the procedure that was performed on a patient and assigns specific diagnoses to that procedure. This data is then entered into the system to assist in generating a patient claim, which is then submitted to the patient's insurance carrier. Ensuring that this information is entered correctly is pivotal to getting timely reimbursements from insurance carriers.

Navigating SimChart

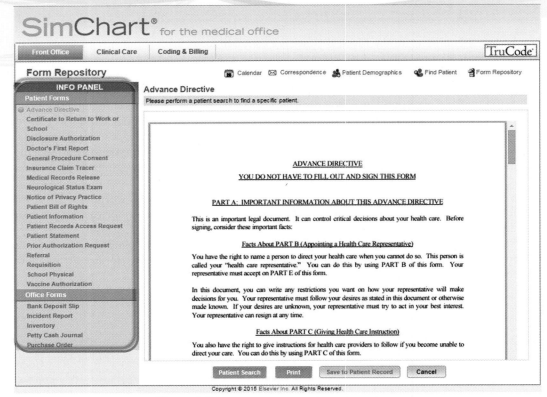

Figure 1-21 Templates in the Form Repository.

Accounting is necessary to keep any office running smoothly and Unit 4 covers the method for tracking payments from both patients and insurance carriers into specific patient ledgers. Whether a patient makes a copayment at the time of the visit or is billed for coinsurance later in the appointment cycle, these payments need to be documented on the correct accounting record in the patient's record. These records need to be accurate so that the office can keep track of the outstanding balances assigned to each patient.

Reporting (Unit 5) is the method by which a practice manager is able to analyze data from a larger perspective to ensure that an office is running smoothly and efficiently. Some reports that are run in a practice can be as simple as a list of patients who are scheduled to be seen on any given day, whereas reports having to do with accounting may be slightly more complex. A Day Sheet is a running log of all payments and charges processed on a given day. In most practices the totals from the day sheet are added to a monthly report that is then used to create a quarterly report, which is then used to create an annual report. The day sheet is one of the major resources used when making financial decisions for the practice. An activity report can track all instances of a specific procedure or diagnosis over a given period. This can be used to build efficiency in the scheduling process, pull out a specific type of patient for follow-up communication, or even order more medical supplies. An aging report lists outstanding charges by how old they are (e.g., 0-30, 60, or 90 days past due). These are used to follow up with patients and insurance carriers that have not made their payments on time, and potentially to send accounts to collections.

The last unit (Unit 6) pulls the entire text together by providing four comprehensive cases beginning with registering new patients for same-day office visits, then coding and submitting claims for each, and finally completing ledgers and day sheets for all relevant payments. All of the individual aspects that had been built up in the previous units will be pulled together to provide the larger picture of how all of the tasks related to a medical office fit together and support each other.

 Now complete the Review Questions for this unit on your Evolve site.

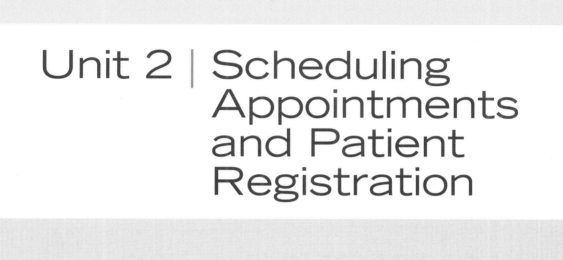

Unit 2 | Scheduling Appointments and Patient Registration

The calendar of a practice can be a useful organization tool. In SimChart for the Medical Office the calendar can be sorted by specific providers or specific examination rooms. The former option is useful when searching out available appointments, or rescheduling a specific block of time for a specific provider. Sorting by exam room is only a useful tool if exam rooms are assigned at the time the patient appointment is set up. For instance, this might be helpful if a patient needs a procedure requiring equipment specific to one room. If an office has one specific room in which a colposcopy can be performed, a practice manager might insist on having that room assigned to all office visits requiring that procedure to ensure that the room is not double booked. Double booking slows down the flow of the office, leading to both unhappy patients and frustrated physicians.

In the Front Office module of SimChart for the Medical Office, appointments can be scheduled one of two ways: (1) clicking on the Add Appointment button, or (2) clicking anywhere within the calendar. Either method will result in a window opening and prompting for more information on the nature of the appointment (Figure 2-1). It is important to ensure that the correct provider is selected for the appointment and, for reasons explained below, the correct amount of time is provided as well.

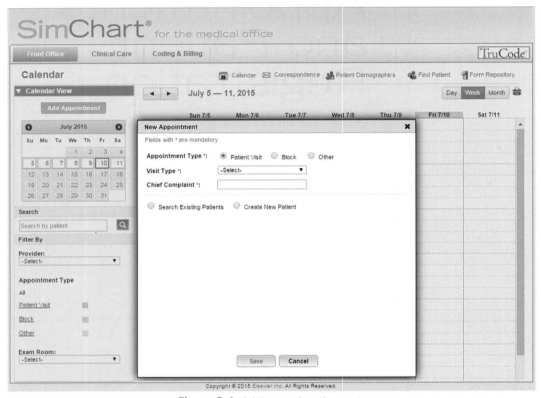

Figure 2-1 Adding an Appointment.

The calendar is used to schedule patient appointments, the first step of the medical office workflow. Both new and existing patients will schedule appointments with a provider for an examination or consultation either as preventative care or to discuss a medical problem. Patient appointments will vary in duration depending on the nature of the patient (new or existing), the nature of the visit, and the comprehensiveness of the diagnosis. For example, a new patient will typically require more time than an existing patient with the same complaint, and a preoperative consultation will typically take longer than a follow-up visit. Each practice has a method for determining these times, and it is important for those scheduling appointments to know the company practice and comply with it. Scheduling too much time for patient visits is not an efficient use of the provider's time and can clog up the schedule, making it difficult for patients to get an appointment in a timely manner. Scheduling too little time can be just as problematic, causing the schedule to get behind and patients to get frustrated as they wait long beyond the time their appointments were scheduled. Finding the right balance and communicating that to the staff is imperative to any practice manager.

New patients also must have their demographic information registered, or input, into the practice management system. This is typically done by having the patient complete a Patient Information

Form, which asks for identifying information (e.g., name, address, phone numbers, insurance) and socioeconomic information (e.g., age, sex, marital status, occupation). Each practice typically develops a Patient Information Form specific to its own needs, sometimes including a bit of health history on the form along with the demographic information. In the case of Walden-Martin Family Medical Clinic, two Patient Information Forms are available: a standard one (Figure 2-2), and one specific to the dental patients of the practice (Figure 2-3). It is possible for a patient to complete two different Patient Information Forms if he or she sees the dentist and one of the other providers of the practice.

WALDEN-MARTIN
FAMILY MEDICAL CLINIC
1234 ANYSTREET | ANYTOWN, ANYSTATE 12345
PHONE 123-123-1234 | FAX 123-123-5678

JULIE WALDEN MD
JAMES MARTIN MD
DAVID KAHN MD
ANGELA PEREZ MD
PATRICK TAYLOR DDS
JEAN BURKE NP

PATIENT INFORMATION

| First Name | MI | Last Name | Date of Birth | Sex |

| SSN | Home Phone | Work Phone | Cell |

| Home Address | City | State | Zip |

| Marital Status | Employer | Driver's License # |

| Emergency Contact | Relationship to Patient | Phone Number |

RESPONSIBLE PARTY INFORMATION   SELF ☐

| First Name | MI | Last Name | Date of Birth | Sex |

| SSN | Home Phone | Work Phone | Cell |

| Home Address | City | State | Zip |

| Employer | Relationship to Patient |

INSURANCE INFORMATION

| Primary Insurance Carrier | Phone Number |

| Address | City | State | Zip |

| Policy Holder Name (if different from patient) | Phone | Date of Birth | Sex |

| Policy Number | Group Number |

| Secondary Insurance Carrier | Phone Number |

| Address | City | State | Zip |

| Policy Holder Name (if different from patient) | Phone | Date of Birth | Sex |

| Policy Number | Group Number |

I hereby give lifetime authorization for payment of insurance benefits to be made directly to Walden-Martin Medical Group, and any assisting physicians, for services rendered. I understand that I am financially responsible for all charges whether or not they are covered by insurance. In the event of default, I agree to pay all costs of collection, and reasonable attorney's fees. I hereby authorize this healthcare provider to release all information necessary to secure the payment of benefits. I further agree that a photocopy of this agreement shall be as valid as the original.

| Signature | Date |

Figure 2-2 Standard Patient Information Form.

Front Office

WALDEN-MARTIN
FAMILY MEDICAL CLINIC
1234 ANYSTREET | ANYTOWN, ANYSTATE 12345
PHONE 123-123-1234 | FAX 123-123-5678

JULIE WALDEN MD
JAMES MARTIN MD
DAVID KAHN MD
ANGELA PEREZ MD
PATRICK TAYLOR DDS
JEAN BURKE NP

DENTAL

PATIENT INFORMATION

First Name	MI	Last Name	Date of Birth	Sex

SSN	Home Phone	Work Phone	Cell

Home Address	City	State	Zip

Marital Status	Employer	Driver's License #

Emergency Contact	Relationship to Patient	Phone Number

RESPONSIBLE PARTY INFORMATION   SELF ☐

First Name	MI	Last Name	Date of Birth	Sex

SSN	Home Phone	Work Phone	Cell

Home Address	City	State	Zip

Employer		Relationship to Patient

DENTAL INSURANCE INFORMATION

Primary Insurance Carrier	Phone Number

Address	City	State	Zip

Policy Holder Name (if different from patient)	Phone	Date of Birth	Sex

Policy Number	Group Number

I hereby give lifetime authorization for payment of insurance benefits to be made directly to Walden-Martin Medical Group, and any assisting physicians, for services rendered. I understand that I am financially responsible for all charges whether or not they are covered by insurance. In the event of default, I agree to pay all costs of collection, and reasonable attorney's fees. I hereby authorize this healthcare provider to release all information necessary to secure the payment of benefits. I further agree that a photocopy of this agreement shall be as valid as the original.

Signature	Date

Figure 2-3 Dental Patient Information Form.

Both of these paper forms are used to input data into the same place: the patient demographics. In SimChart for the Medical Office this can be accessed by clicking on the common icon titled Patient Demographics at the top of the screen (Figure 2-4). There are three tabs (Patient, Guarantor, and Insurance) with fields that can be filled in using the information from the Patient Information Form submitted by the patient. Some fields are mandatory to save the patient in the system, whereas others include information that might be useful but not critical. Once patients are set up via the Patient Demographics tool they can then be scheduled for appointments and have their encounters documented and billed.

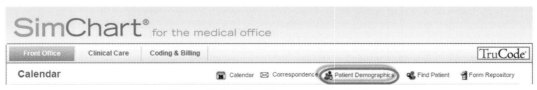

Figure 2-4 Patient Demographics Tool.

Scheduling an Appointment for an Existing Patient

Quinton Brown (DOB 02/24/1978) is calling the Walden-Martin Family Medical Clinic to request a follow-up visit with Dr. Martin. He recently was diagnosed with pneumonia and given a round of antibiotics. He was instructed to take all the antibiotics and then schedule a follow-up appointment with Dr. Martin. Because this is a follow-up appointment to ensure that the round of antibiotics worked, this appointment should be fifteen minutes. Mr. Brown would like an appointment sometime next Thursday afternoon.

Measurable Steps

1. Within the Calendar of the Front Office module, click the Add Appointment button (Figure 2-5) or click anywhere within the calendar to open the New Appointment window.

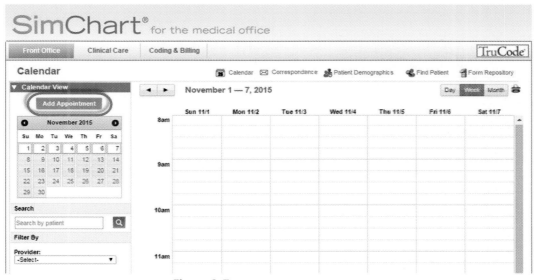

Figure 2-5 Add Appointment button.

2. Select the Patient Visit radio button as the Appointment Type.
3. Select Follow-Up/Established from the Visit Type dropdown.

◎ **HELPFUL HINT**

A brief description of visit types is as follows:
- Annual Exam: A patient visit that occurs yearly and includes a complete physical examination.
- Comprehensive: A patient visit that includes a complex medical diagnosis and will require more time than a typical exam.
- Follow-Up/Established: Patient visit for a patient following up on a previously diagnosed condition or a patient who has been seen in the medical office within the last three years but is not coming in for an annual exam, urgent visit, or wellness exam.
- New Patient: A patient who is seeing the physician for the first time or who has not been to the medical office within the last three years.

Continued

HELPFUL HINT—cont'd

- Urgent: Patient visit type for a patient with a serious condition who must see the physician on the same day they request an appointment.
- Wellness Exam: This visit type encompasses preventive services such as a colonoscopy, sigmoidoscopy, mammogram, or bone density study.
- 6-Month Visit: This visit type is specific to dental patients and encompasses regular 6-month cleanings.

4. Document "Pneumonia follow-up" in the Chief Complaint text box.
5. Select the Search Existing Patients radio button.
6. Using the Patient Search fields, search for Mr. Brown's patient record. Once you locate Mr. Brown in the List of Patients, confirm his date of birth (Figure 2-6).

HELPFUL HINT

Confirming date of birth will help to ensure that you have located the correct patient record.

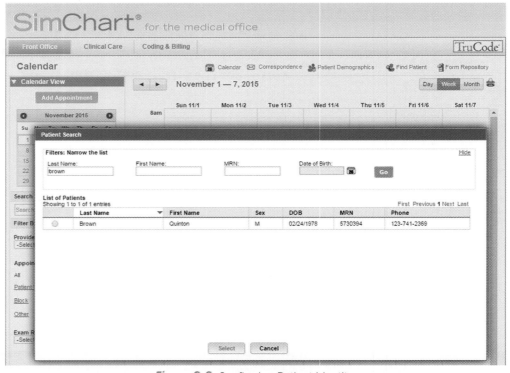

Figure 2-6 Confirming Patient Identity.

7. Select the radio button for Quinton Brown and click the Select button. Confirm the autopopulated details.
8. Select the correct provider from the Provider dropdown menu.
9. Use the calendar picker to confirm or select the appointment day.
10. Select a start and end time for the appointment using the Start Time and End Time dropdowns.
11. Click the Save button. A confirmation message will appear.
12. Click the OK button to proceed.
13. Mr. Brown's appointment will appear on the calendar (Figure 2-7).

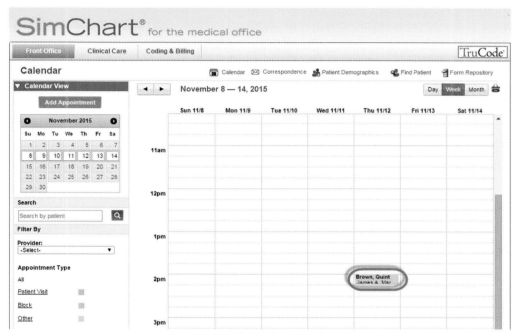

Figure 2-7 Patient Appointment in the Calendar.

Activity

Now schedule the following appointments for existing patients at Walden-Martin Family Medical Clinic:

Patient	DOB	Date and Duration of Service	Chief Complaint	Visit Type
Dr. Walden				
Walter Biller	01/04/1970	Next Thursday Afternoon (30 minutes)	Wellness Exam	Wellness Exam
Erma Willis	12/09/1947	Next Tuesday Morning (15 minutes)	adenocarcinoma	Follow up/ Established
Dr. Martin				
Isabella Burgel	07/23/2010	Next Wednesday Morning (15 minutes)	Down syndrome	Follow up/ Established
Pedro Gomez	07/01/2007	Next Monday Afternoon (15 minutes)	Flu	Follow up/ Established
Maude Crawford	12/22/1946	Next Friday Morning (30 minutes)	Annual Exam	Annual Exam
Jean Burke				
Tai Yan	04/07/1956	Next Thursday Morning (30 minutes)	Annual Exam	Annual Exam
Johnny Parker	06/15/2010	Next Tuesday Afternoon (1 hour)	Wellness Exam	Wellness Exam
Dr. Taylor				
Noemi Rodriguez	11/04/1971	Next Monday Afternoon (30 minutes)	Teeth cleaning	6 Month Visit
Reuven Ahmad	09/12/1967	Next Friday Afternoon (30 minutes)	Teeth cleaning	6 Month Visit
Dr. Perez				
Truong Tran	05/30/1991	Next Wednesday Afternoon (15 minutes)	Chronic Heartburn	Follow up/ Established
Kyle Reeves	01/01/1996	Next Friday Morning (30 minutes)	Abdominal pain	Follow up/ Established
Jana Green	05/01/1936	Next Thursday Afternoon (30 minutes)	Irritable bowel Syndrome	Follow up/ Established
Dr. Kahn				
Monique Jones	06/23/1985	Next Tuesday Morning (45 minutes)	Rash	Comprehensive Visit

Registering a New Patient

Maddy Martin (DOB 03/12/1983) wants to schedule a new patient visit with Dr. Kahn. She has a family history of skin cancer and would like to begin regular checkups with a dermatologist. She has a few specific spots that concern her, but would like an overall evaluation also for peace of mind. To mitigate the amount of paperwork she will need to do in the office, she asked you to fax her the patient information form and she has faxed her completed patient information form and insurance card (Figure 2-8) to Walden-Martin Family Medical Clinic this morning. She is awaiting a call from Dr. Kahn's office regarding an appointment date and time.

WALDEN-MARTIN
FAMILY MEDICAL CLINIC
1234 ANYSTREET | ANYTOWN, ANYSTATE 12345
PHONE 123-123-1234 | FAX 123-123-5678

JULIE WALDEN MD
JAMES MARTIN MD
DAVID KAHN MD
ANGELA PEREZ MD
PATRICK TAYLOR DDS
JEAN BURKE NP

PATIENT INFORMATION

First Name	MI	Last Name	Date of Birth	Sex
Maddy	S	Martin	3/12/1983	F

SSN	Home Phone	Work Phone	Cell
758-27-4239	123-262-8867		

Home Address	City	State	Zip
4476 Wright Way	Anytown	AL	12345-1234

Marital Status	Employer	Driver's License #
Single	Anytown Bank	WQ56059030

Emergency Contact	Relationship to Patient	Phone Number
Dorothy Thick		123-335-2871

RESPONSIBLE PARTY INFORMATION SELF ☑

First Name	MI	Last Name	Date of Birth	Sex
Maddy	S	Martin	3/12/1983	F

SSN	Home Phone	Work Phone	Cell
758-27-4239	123-262-8867		

Home Address	City	State	Zip
4476 Wright Way	Anytown	AL	12345-1234

Employer		Relationship to Patient
Anytown Bank		Self

INSURANCE INFORMATION

Primary Insurance Carrier	Phone Number
Aetna	1-800-123-2222

Address	City	State	Zip
1234 Insurance Way	Anytown	AL	12345-1234

Policy Holder Name (if different from patient)	Phone	Date of Birth	Sex

Policy Number	Group Number	
GD1683162	12548M	

Secondary Insurance Carrier	Phone Number

Address	City	State	Zip

Policy Holder Name (if different from patient)	Phone	Date of Birth	Sex

Policy Number	Group Number	

I hereby give lifetime authorization for payment of insurance benefits to be made directly to Walden-Martin Medical Group, and any assisting physicians, for services rendered. I understand that I am financially responsible for all charges whether or not they are covered by insurance. In the event of default, I agree to pay all costs of collection, and reasonable attorney's fees. I hereby authorize this healthcare provider to release all information necessary to secure the payment of benefits. I further agree that a photocopy of this agreement shall be as valid as the original.

Signature	Date
Maddy S. Martin	

AETNA 1234 Insurance Way

MEMBER NAME: Martin, Maddy

POLICY #: GD1683162
GROUP #: 12548M

DEPENDENTS:
EFFECTIVE DATE:
08/24/2015

CO-PAY: $25
SPECIALIST CO-PAY: $50
ER: $200

DRUG CO-PAY
GENERIC: $10
NAME BRAND: $50

Member Services: 1-800-123-2222

Figure 2-8 Maddy Martin Patient Information Form and Insurance Card.

1. Click the Patient Demographics icon (Figure 2-9).

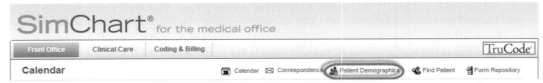

Figure 2-9 Patient Demographics.

2. Perform a patient search to confirm that Maddy Martin is not an existing patient.
3. Click the Add Patient button (Figure 2-10).

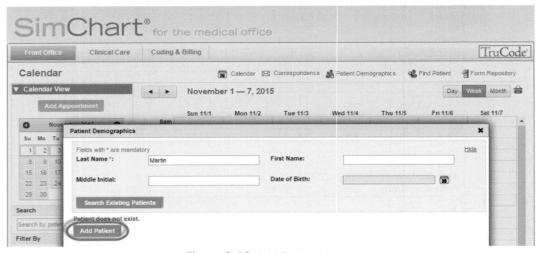

Figure 2-10 Add Patient button.

4. Using the completed patient information form and insurance card as reference, complete the following fields in the Patient tab: Last Name, First Name, Middle Initial, Date of Birth (Age will autopopulate from this), Sex, SSN, Emergency Contact, Emergency Contact Phone, Address, City, Country, State, and Zip/Postal Code.
5. Select the Guarantor tab (see Helpful Hint below for more details on Guarantors). Because Maddy is on her own insurance plan, select the radio button next to Self. Most of the information from the Patient tab will populate this tab. Make sure to fill in the Employer and select the correct provider.

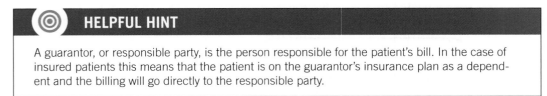

HELPFUL HINT

A guarantor, or responsible party, is the person responsible for the patient's bill. In the case of insured patients this means that the patient is on the guarantor's insurance plan as a dependent and the billing will go directly to the responsible party.

6. Select the Insurance tab. Select the correct insurance carrier from the dropdown menu and the correct address and phone number should autopopulate. Complete the remaining fields in the Primary Insurance tab and click the Save Patient button to save Maddy Martin's demographic information (Figure 2-11).

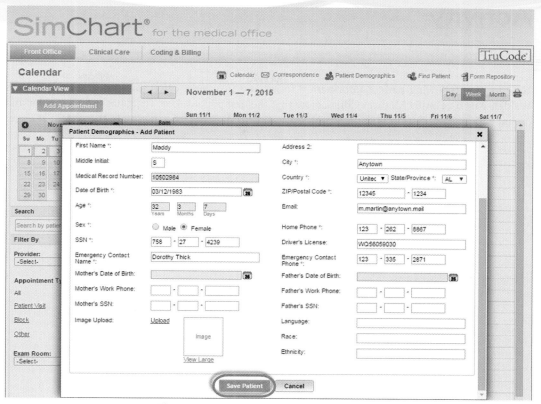

Figure 2-11 Saving Patient Demographics.

7. A confirmation message will appear (Figure 2-12). If you are finished inputting data, click the Yes button. You will automatically be redirected to Maddy Martin's patient record.

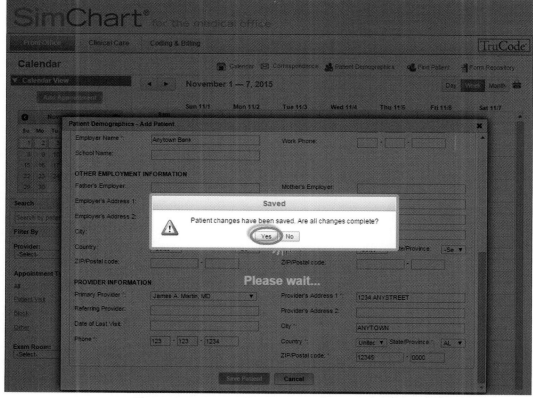

Figure 2-12 Confirmation of Patient Demographics.

Activity

Now use the following patient information forms and insurance cards to register new patients to Walden-Martin Family Medical Clinic. Note that the first patient, Lou Thao, has both a regular and dental Patient Information Form. Use both to complete all of his information in the system at once.

WALDEN-MARTIN
FAMILY MEDICAL CLINIC
1234 ANYSTREET | ANYTOWN, ANYSTATE 12345
PHONE 123-123-1234 | FAX 123-123-5678

JULIE WALDEN MD
JAMES MARTIN MD
DAVID KAHN MD
ANGELA PEREZ MD
PATRICK TAYLOR DDS
JEAN BURKE NP

PATIENT INFORMATION

First Name	MI	Last Name	Date of Birth	Sex
Lou		Thao	11/27/72	M

SSN	Home Phone	Work Phone	Cell
783-73-3398	123-627-4851		

Home Address	City	State	Zip
380 Bunsen Way	Anytown	AL	12345-1234

Marital Status	Employer	Driver's License #
Married	Anytown Bar and Grill	EF74635896

Emergency Contact	Relationship to Patient	Phone Number
May Thao	Wife	123-627-5784

RESPONSIBLE PARTY INFORMATION   SELF ☑

First Name	MI	Last Name	Date of Birth	Sex
Lou		Thao	11/27/72	M

SSN	Home Phone	Work Phone	Cell
783-73-3398	123-627-4851		

Home Address	City	State	Zip
380 Bunsen Way	Anytown	AL	12345-1234

Employer		Relationship to Patient
Anytown Bar and Grill		Self

INSURANCE INFORMATION

Primary Insurance Carrier	Phone Number
Aetna	1-800-123-2222

Address	City	State	Zip
1234 Insurance Way	Anytown	AL	12345-1234

Policy Holder Name (if different from patient)	Phone	Date of Birth	Sex

Policy Number	Group Number
ZT3077974	81407W

Secondary Insurance Carrier	Phone Number

Address	City	State	Zip

Policy Holder Name (if different from patient)	Phone	Date of Birth	Sex

Policy Number	Group Number

I hereby give lifetime authorization for payment of insurance benefits to be made directly to Walden-Martin Medical Group, and any assisting physicians, for services rendered. I understand that I am financially responsible for all charges whether or not they are covered by insurance. In the event of default, I agree to pay all costs of collection, and reasonable attorney's fees. I hereby authorize this healthcare provider to release all information necessary to secure the payment of benefits. I further agree that a photocopy of this agreement shall be as valid as the original.

Signature *Lou Thao*	Date

AETNA   **1234 Insurance Way**

MEMBER NAME: Thao, Lou

POLICY #: ZT3077974   **DEPENDENTS:**
GROUP #: 81407W   **EFFECTIVE DATE:**
                                      08/24/2015

CO-PAY: $25   DRUG CO-PAY:
SPECIALIST CO-PAY: $50   GENERIC: $10
ER: $200   NAME BRAND: $50

Member Services: 1-800-123-2222

WALDEN-MARTIN
FAMILY MEDICAL CLINIC
1234 ANYSTREET | ANYTOWN, ANYSTATE 12345
PHONE 123-123-1234 | FAX 123-123-5678

JULIE WALDEN MD
JAMES MARTIN MD
DAVID KAHN MD
ANGELA PEREZ MD
PATRICK TAYLOR DDS
JEAN BURKE NP

DENTAL

PATIENT INFORMATION

First Name	MI	Last Name	Date of Birth	Sex
Lou		Thao	11/27/72	M

SSN	Home Phone	Work Phone	Cell
783-73-3398	123-627-4851		

Home Address	City	State	Zip
380 Bunsen Way	Anytown	AL	12345-1234

Marital Status	Employer	Driver's License #
Married	Anytown Bar and Grill	EF74635896

Emergency Contact	Relationship to Patient	Phone Number
May Thao	Wife	123-627-5784

RESPONSIBLE PARTY INFORMATION   SELF ☑

First Name	MI	Last Name	Date of Birth	Sex
Lou		Thao	11/27/72	M

SSN	Home Phone	Work Phone	Cell
783-73-3398	123-627-4851		

Home Address	City	State	Zip
380 Bunsen Way	Anytown	AL	12345-1234

Employer		Relationship to Patient
Anytown Bar and Grill		Self

DENTAL INSURANCE INFORMATION

Primary Insurance Carrier	Phone Number
Aetna PPO (Dental)	1-800-123-3434

Address	City	State	Zip
1234 Insurance Way	Anytown	AL	12345-1234

Policy Holder Name (if different from patient)	Phone	Date of Birth	Sex

Policy Number	Group Number
UN986456	81407D

I hereby give lifetime authorization for payment of insurance benefits to be made directly to Walden-Martin Medical Group, and any assisting physicians, for services rendered. I understand that I am financially responsible for all charges whether or not they are covered by insurance. In the event of default, I agree to pay all costs of collection, and reasonable attorney's fees. I hereby authorize this healthcare provider to release all information necessary to secure the payment of benefits. I further agree that a photocopy of this agreement shall be as valid as the original.

Signature	Date
Lou Thao	

AETNA DENTAL PPO   **1234 Insurance Way**

MEMBER NAME: Thao, Lou

POLICY #: UN986456   DEPENDENTS:
GROUP #: 81407D   EFFECTIVE DATE: 06/01/2015

Member Services: 1-800-123-2222

WALDEN-MARTIN
FAMILY MEDICAL CLINIC
1234 ANYSTREET | ANYTOWN, ANYSTATE 12345
PHONE 123-123-1234 | FAX 123-123-5678

JULIE WALDEN MD
JAMES MARTIN MD
DAVID KAHN MD
ANGELA PEREZ MD
PATRICK TAYLOR DDS
JEAN BURKE NP

PATIENT INFORMATION

First Name	MI	Last Name	Date of Birth	Sex
Boyd	C	Dubois	4/30/1958	M

SSN	Home Phone	Work Phone	Cell
561-83-8750	123-721-2131		

Home Address	City	State	Zip
62 Little Flock Rd.	Anytown	AL	12345-1234

Marital Status	Employer	Driver's License #
Married	Anytown Factory	JS11486688

Emergency Contact	Relationship to Patient	Phone Number
Betty Dubois		123-721-2131

RESPONSIBLE PARTY INFORMATION   SELF ☑

First Name	MI	Last Name	Date of Birth	Sex
Boyd	C	Dubois	4/30/1958	M

SSN	Home Phone	Work Phone	Cell
561-83-8750	123-721-2131		

Home Address	City	State	Zip
62 Little Flock Rd.	Anytown	AL	12345-1234

Employer		Relationship to Patient
Anytown Factory		Self

INSURANCE INFORMATION

Primary Insurance Carrier	Phone Number
Total Medical Insurance	1-800-123-1212

Address	City	State	Zip
1255 Insurance Avenue	Anytown	AL	12345-1234

Policy Holder Name (if different from patient)	Phone	Date of Birth	Sex

Policy Number	Group Number	
MW3693268	79521P	

Secondary Insurance Carrier	Phone Number

Address	City	State	Zip

Policy Holder Name (if different from patient)	Phone	Date of Birth	Sex

Policy Number	Group Number

I hereby give lifetime authorization for payment of insurance benefits to be made directly to Walden-Martin Medical Group, and any assisting physicians, for services rendered. I understand that I am financially responsible for all charges whether or not they are covered by insurance. In the event of default, I agree to pay all costs of collection, and reasonable attorney's fees. I hereby authorize this healthcare provider to release all information necessary to secure the payment of benefits. I further agree that a photocopy of this agreement shall be as valid as the original.

Signature *Boyd C. Dubois*	Date

Total Medical Insurance

MEMBER NAME: Dubois, Boyd

POLICY NUMBER: MW3693268
GROUP #: 79521P
DEPENDENTS:

EFFECTIVE DATE:
07/27/2015

CO-PAY: $25
SPECIALIST CO-PAY: $50
ER: $250

DRUG CO-PAY
GENERIC: $20
NAME BRAND: $40

CLAIMS/INQUIRIES: 1-800-123-1212

WALDEN-MARTIN
FAMILY MEDICAL CLINIC
1234 ANYSTREET | ANYTOWN, ANYSTATE 12345
PHONE 123-123-1234 | FAX 123-123-5678

JULIE WALDEN MD
JAMES MARTIN MD
DAVID KAHN MD
ANGELA PEREZ MD
PATRICK TAYLOR DDS
JEAN BURKE NP

PATIENT INFORMATION

First Name	MI	Last Name	Date of Birth	Sex
Jessie		Baer	5/25/1995	F

SSN	Home Phone	Work Phone	Cell
567-27-3938	123-555-7654		

Home Address	City	State	Zip
6749 W. Eastend Ave.	Anytown	AL	12345-1234

Marital Status	Employer	Driver's License #
Single	Anytown Coffee	KE80148639

Emergency Contact	Relationship to Patient	Phone Number
Elan Lonata		123-555-9878

RESPONSIBLE PARTY INFORMATION   SELF ☑

First Name	MI	Last Name	Date of Birth	Sex
Jessie		Baer	5/25/1995	F

SSN	Home Phone	Work Phone	Cell
567-27-3938	123-555-7654		

Home Address	City	State	Zip
6749 W. Eastend Ave.	Anytown	AL	12345-1234

Employer		Relationship to Patient
Anytown Coffee		Self

INSURANCE INFORMATION

Primary Insurance Carrier	Phone Number
Helping Hand	1-800-123-8888

Address	City	State	Zip
1255 Insurance Way	Anytown	AL	12345-1234

Policy Holder Name (if different from patient)	Phone	Date of Birth	Sex

Policy Number	Group Number
NJ6722142	76100J

Secondary Insurance Carrier	Phone Number

Address	City	State	Zip

Policy Holder Name (if different from patient)	Phone	Date of Birth	Sex

Policy Number	Group Number

I hereby give lifetime authorization for payment of insurance benefits to be made directly to Walden-Martin Medical Group, and any assisting physicians, for services rendered. I understand that I am financially responsible for all charges whether or not they are covered by insurance. In the event of default, I agree to pay all costs of collection, and reasonable attorney's fees. I hereby authorize this healthcare provider to release all information necessary to secure the payment of benefits. I further agree that a photocopy of this agreement shall be as valid as the original.

Signature	Date
Jessie Bauer	

Helping Hand

MEMBER NAME: Baer, Jessie   **EFFECTIVE DATE:** 11/24/2015
POLICY NUMBER: NJ6722142
GROUP #: 76100J
DEPENDENTS:

Network Coinsurance: DRUG CO-PAY
In: 75% / 25%   GENERIC: $10
Out: 50% / 50%   NAME BRAND: $40

CLAIMS/INQUIRIES: 1-800-123-8888

WALDEN-MARTIN
FAMILY MEDICAL CLINIC
1234 ANYSTREET | ANYTOWN, ANYSTATE 12345
PHONE 123-123-1234 | FAX 123-123-5678

JULIE WALDEN MD
JAMES MARTIN MD
DAVID KAHN MD
ANGELA PEREZ MD
PATRICK TAYLOR DDS
JEAN BURKE NP

DENTAL

PATIENT INFORMATION

First Name	MI	Last Name	Date of Birth	Sex
Kim		Nguyen	10/1/54	F

SSN	Home Phone	Work Phone	Cell
392-06-2329	123-321-2841		

Home Address	City	State	Zip
4853 S. Maple St.	Anytown	AL	12345-1234

Marital Status	Employer	Driver's License #
Widowed	Anytown Diner	AQ50262118

Emergency Contact	Relationship to Patient	Phone Number
Sue Ann Wilson	Daughter	123-485-1825

RESPONSIBLE PARTY INFORMATION   SELF ☑

First Name	MI	Last Name	Date of Birth	Sex
Kim		Nguyen	10/1/54	F

SSN	Home Phone	Work Phone	Cell
392-06-2329	123-321-2841		

Home Address	City	State	Zip
4853 S. Maple St.	Anytown	AL	12345-1234

Employer		Relationship to Patient
Anytown Diner		Self

DENTAL INSURANCE INFORMATION

Primary Insurance Carrier	Phone Number
Delta Dental DMO	1-800-123-4545

Address	City	State	Zip
1255 Insurance Boulevard	Anytown	AL	12345-1234

Policy Holder Name (if different from patient)	Phone	Date of Birth	Sex

Policy Number	Group Number	
CJ7455924	259845T	

I hereby give lifetime authorization for payment of insurance benefits to be made directly to Walden-Martin Medical Group, and any assisting physicians, for services rendered. I understand that I am financially responsible for all charges whether or not they are covered by insurance. In the event of default, I agree to pay all costs of collection, and reasonable attorney's fees. I hereby authorize this healthcare provider to release all information necessary to secure the payment of benefits. I further agree that a photocopy of this agreement shall be as valid as the original.

Signature	Date
Kim Nguyen	

Delta Dental   DMO

MEMBER NAME: Nguyen, Kim

POLICY NUMBER: CJ7455924
GROUP #: 259845T   **EFFECTIVE DATE:**
DEPENDENTS: 06/01/2015

CLAIMS/INQUIRIES: 1-800-123-4545

WALDEN-MARTIN
FAMILY MEDICAL CLINIC
1234 ANYSTREET | ANYTOWN, ANYSTATE 12345
PHONE 123-123-1234 | FAX 123-123-5678

JULIE WALDEN MD
JAMES MARTIN MD
DAVID KAHN MD
ANGELA PEREZ MD
PATRICK TAYLOR DDS
JEAN BURKE NP

PATIENT INFORMATION

First Name	MI	Last Name	Date of Birth	Sex
Dee	T	Falcione	6/12/1981	M

SSN	Home Phone	Work Phone	Cell
712-79-5715	123-897-1572		

Home Address	City	State	Zip
12 Windjammer Rd.	Anytown	AL	12345-1234

Marital Status	Employer	Driver's License #
Single	Anytown Supermarket	DJ50483440

Emergency Contact	Relationship to Patient	Phone Number
Mary Falcione	Mother	123-897-1572

RESPONSIBLE PARTY INFORMATION   SELF ☑

First Name	MI	Last Name	Date of Birth	Sex
Dee	T	Falcione	6/12/1981	M

SSN	Home Phone	Work Phone	Cell
712-79-5715	123-897-1572		

Home Address	City	State	Zip
12 Windjammer Rd.	Anytown	AL	12345-1234

Employer		Relationship to Patient
Anytown Supermarket		Self

INSURANCE INFORMATION

Primary Insurance Carrier	Phone Number
Western Health	1-800-123-2323

Address	City	State	Zip
1255 Insurance Place	Anytown	AL	12345-1234

Policy Holder Name (if different from patient)	Phone	Date of Birth	Sex

Policy Number	Group Number
KR1170991	79426B

Secondary Insurance Carrier	Phone Number

Address	City	State	Zip

Policy Holder Name (if different from patient)	Phone	Date of Birth	Sex

Policy Number	Group Number

I hereby give lifetime authorization for payment of insurance benefits to be made directly to Walden-Martin Medical Group, and any assisting physicians, for services rendered. I understand that I am financially responsible for all charges whether or not they are covered by insurance. In the event of default, I agree to pay all costs of collection, and reasonable attorney's fees. I hereby authorize this healthcare provider to release all information necessary to secure the payment of benefits. I further agree that a photocopy of this agreement shall be as valid as the original.

Signature *Dee T. Falcione*	Date

Western Health

MEMBER NAME: Falcione, Dee

POLICY NUMBER: KR1170991
GROUP #: 79426B
DEPENDENTS:

EFFECTIVE DATE:
10/01/2015

CO-PAY: $25
SPECIALIST CO-PAY: $35
XRAY/LAB BENEFIT: $250

DRUG CO-PAY
GENERIC: $10
NAME BRAND: $50

CLAIMS/INQUIRIES: 1-800-123-1212

WALDEN-MARTIN
FAMILY MEDICAL CLINIC
1234 ANYSTREET | ANYTOWN, ANYSTATE 12345
PHONE 123-123-1234 | FAX 123-123-5678

JULIE WALDEN MD
JAMES MARTIN MD
DAVID KAHN MD
ANGELA PEREZ MD
PATRICK TAYLOR DDS
JEAN BURKE NP

PATIENT INFORMATION

First Name	MI	Last Name		Date of Birth	Sex
Jesus		Garcia		9/9/1988	M

SSN	Home Phone	Work Phone		Cell
985-97-8567	123-555-1444			

Home Address	City	State	Zip
1234 Miller Rd.	Anytown	AL	12345-1234

Marital Status	Employer	Driver's License #
Single	Anytown Construction	EY53329861

Emergency Contact	Relationship to Patient	Phone Number
Virginia Jones		123-555-1212

RESPONSIBLE PARTY INFORMATION   SELF ☑

First Name	MI	Last Name		Date of Birth	Sex
Jesus		Garcia		9/9/1988	M

SSN	Home Phone	Work Phone		Cell
985-97-8567	123-555-1444			

Home Address	City	State	Zip
1234 Miller Rd.	Anytown	AL	12345-1234

Employer		Relationship to Patient
Anytown Construction		Self

INSURANCE INFORMATION

Primary Insurance Carrier	Phone Number
MetLife	1-800-123-4444

Address	City	State	Zip
1234 Insurance Avenue	Anytown	AL	12345-1234

Policy Holder Name (if different from patient)	Phone	Date of Birth	Sex

Policy Number	Group Number	
CY2593928	63885K	

Secondary Insurance Carrier	Phone Number

Address	City	State	Zip

Policy Holder Name (if different from patient)	Phone	Date of Birth	Sex

Policy Number	Group Number	

I hereby give lifetime authorization for payment of insurance benefits to be made directly to Walden-Martin Medical Group, and any assisting physicians, for services rendered. I understand that I am financially responsible for all charges whether or not they are covered by insurance. In the event of default, I agree to pay all costs of collection, and reasonable attorney's fees. I hereby authorize this healthcare provider to release all information necessary to secure the payment of benefits. I further agree that a photocopy of this agreement shall be as valid as the original.

Signature *Jesus Garcia*	Date

MetLife   1234 Insurance Avenue

MEMBER NAME: Garcia, Jesus

POLICY #: CY2593928
GROUP #: 63885K   **EFFECTIVE DATE:**
                                    08/24/2015

CO-PAY: $25   DRUG CO-PAY
SPECIALIST CO-PAY: $35   GENERIC: $15
XRAY/LAB BENEFIT: $250   NAME BRAND: $30

CLAIMS/INQUIRIES: 1-800-123-4444

WALDEN-MARTIN
FAMILY MEDICAL CLINIC
1234 ANYSTREET | ANYTOWN, ANYSTATE 12345
PHONE 123-123-1234 | FAX 123-123-5678

JULIE WALDEN MD
JAMES MARTIN MD
DAVID KAHN MD
ANGELA PEREZ MD
PATRICK TAYLOR DDS
JEAN BURKE NP

DENTAL

PATIENT INFORMATION

First Name	MI	Last Name	Date of Birth	Sex
Patricia	A	Higgins	5/8/41	F

SSN	Home Phone	Work Phone	Cell
982-77-9510	123-667-4823		

Home Address	City	State	Zip
1242 Mason Lane	Anytown	AL	12345-1234

Marital Status	Employer	Driver's License #
Married	Retired	KE24391368

Emergency Contact	Relationship to Patient	Phone Number
Harold Higgins	Husband	123-667-4823

RESPONSIBLE PARTY INFORMATION   SELF ☑

First Name	MI	Last Name	Date of Birth	Sex
Patricia	A	Higgins	5/8/41	F

SSN	Home Phone	Work Phone	Cell
982-77-9510	123-667-4823		

Home Address	City	State	Zip
1242 Mason Lane	Anytown	AL	12345-1234

Employer		Relationship to Patient
Retired		Self

DENTAL INSURANCE INFORMATION

Primary Insurance Carrier	Phone Number
Medicare (Dental)	1-800-123-3333

Address	City	State	Zip
1234 Insurance Road	Anytown	AL	12345-1234

Policy Holder Name (if different from patient)	Phone	Date of Birth	Sex

Policy Number	Group Number	
734370909A		

I hereby give lifetime authorization for payment of insurance benefits to be made directly to Walden-Martin Medical Group, and any assisting physicians, for services rendered. I understand that I am financially responsible for all charges whether or not they are covered by insurance. In the event of default, I agree to pay all costs of collection, and reasonable attorney's fees. I hereby authorize this healthcare provider to release all information necessary to secure the payment of benefits. I further agree that a photocopy of this agreement shall be as valid as the original.

Signature	Date
Patricia Higgins	

MEDICARE Dental   1234 Insurance Road

MEMBER NAME: Higgins, Patricia

POLICY #: 734370909A
EFFECTIVE DATE: 3/20/2015

Is entitled to:
HOSPITAL   (PART A)
MEDICAL   (PART B)

CLAIMS/INQUIRIES: 1-800-123-3333

WALDEN-MARTIN
FAMILY MEDICAL CLINIC
1234 ANYSTREET | ANYTOWN, ANYSTATE 12345
PHONE 123-123-1234 | FAX 123-123-5678

JULIE WALDEN MD
JAMES MARTIN MD
DAVID KAHN MD
ANGELA PEREZ MD
PATRICK TAYLOR DDS
JEAN BURKE NP

PATIENT INFORMATION

First Name	MI	Last Name	Date of Birth	Sex
Mathias	S	Hedding	1/18/1953	M

SSN	Home Phone	Work Phone	Cell
137-62-8041	123-854-9325		

Home Address	City	State	Zip
3111 N. Cooper St.	Anytown	AL	12345-1234

Marital Status	Employer	Driver's License #
Single	Anytown Supermarket	FJ71976083

Emergency Contact	Relationship to Patient	Phone Number
James Hedding	Cousin	123-741-8529

RESPONSIBLE PARTY INFORMATION   SELF ☑

First Name	MI	Last Name	Date of Birth	Sex
Mathias	S	Hedding	1/18/1953	M

SSN	Home Phone	Work Phone	Cell
137-62-8041	123-854-9325		

Home Address	City	State	Zip
3111 N. Cooper St.	Anytown	AL	12345-1234

Employer		Relationship to Patient
Anytown Supermarket		Self

INSURANCE INFORMATION

Primary Insurance Carrier	Phone Number
None. Self-pay	

Address	City	State	Zip

Policy Holder Name (if different from patient)	Phone	Date of Birth	Sex

Policy Number	Group Number

Secondary Insurance Carrier	Phone Number

Address	City	State	Zip

Policy Holder Name (if different from patient)	Phone	Date of Birth	Sex

Policy Number	Group Number

I hereby give lifetime authorization for payment of insurance benefits to be made directly to Walden-Martin Medical Group, and any assisting physicians, for services rendered. I understand that I am financially responsible for all charges whether or not they are covered by insurance. In the event of default, I agree to pay all costs of collection, and reasonable attorney's fees. I hereby authorize this healthcare provider to release all information necessary to secure the payment of benefits. I further agree that a photocopy of this agreement shall be as valid as the original.

Signature	Date
Mathias S. Hedding	

WALDEN-MARTIN
FAMILY MEDICAL CLINIC
1234 ANYSTREET | ANYTOWN, ANYSTATE 12345
PHONE 123-123-1234 | FAX 123-123-5678

JULIE WALDEN MD
JAMES MARTIN MD
DAVID KAHN MD
ANGELA PEREZ MD
PATRICK TAYLOR DDS
JEAN BURKE NP

PATIENT INFORMATION

First Name	MI	Last Name	Date of Birth	Sex
Robert		Jackson	2/24/1958	M

SSN	Home Phone	Work Phone	Cell
719-19-6141	123-454-3344		

Home Address	City	State	Zip
5647 E. Westlake Road	Anytown	AL	12345-1234

Marital Status	Employer	Driver's License #
Divorced	Unemployed	NW73770847

Emergency Contact	Relationship to Patient	Phone Number
Mary Ann Owen		555-553-4244

RESPONSIBLE PARTY INFORMATION   SELF ☑

First Name	MI	Last Name	Date of Birth	Sex
Robert		Jackson	2/24/1958	M

SSN	Home Phone	Work Phone	Cell
719-19-6141	123-454-3344		

Home Address	City	State	Zip
5647 E. Westlake Road	Anytown	AL	12345-1234

Employer		Relationship to Patient
Unemployed		Self

INSURANCE INFORMATION

Primary Insurance Carrier	Phone Number
Blue Cross/Blue Shield	1-800-123-1111

Address	City	State	Zip
1234 Insurance Place	Anytown	AL	12345-1234

Policy Holder Name (if different from patient)	Phone	Date of Birth	Sex

Policy Number	Group Number
GY2873943	62308A

Secondary Insurance Carrier	Phone Number

Address	City	State	Zip

Policy Holder Name (if different from patient)	Phone	Date of Birth	Sex

Policy Number	Group Number

I hereby give lifetime authorization for payment of insurance benefits to be made directly to Walden-Martin Medical Group, and any assisting physicians, for services rendered. I understand that I am financially responsible for all charges whether or not they are covered by insurance. In the event of default, I agree to pay all costs of collection, and reasonable attorney's fees. I hereby authorize this healthcare provider to release all information necessary to secure the payment of benefits. I further agree that a photocopy of this agreement shall be as valid as the original.

Signature *Robert Jackson*	Date

BLUE CROSS BLUE SHIELD   1234 Insurance Place

MEMBER NAME: Jackson, Robert

DEPENDENT: POLICY #: GY2873943
GROUP #: 62308A   EFFECTIVE DATE:
                             10/13/2015

CO-PAY: $25   Care RX:
SPECIALIST CO-PAY: $35   Rx Bin: 840513
XRAY/LAB BENEFIT: $250   Rx Group: 6410RX

CLAIMS/INQUIRIES: 1-800-123-1111

Front Office

WALDEN-MARTIN
FAMILY MEDICAL CLINIC
1234 ANYSTREET | ANYTOWN, ANYSTATE 12345
PHONE 123-123-1234 | FAX 123-123-5678

JULIE WALDEN MD
JAMES MARTIN MD
DAVID KAHN MD
ANGELA PEREZ MD
PATRICK TAYLOR DDS
JEAN BURKE NP

DENTAL

PATIENT INFORMATION

First Name	MI	Last Name		Date of Birth	Sex
Aaron	T	Logan		6/21/99	M

SSN	Home Phone	Work Phone		Cell
853-18-6583	123-851-1061			

Home Address	City	State	Zip
1412 Gina Dr	Anytown	AL	12345-1234

Marital Status	Employer	Driver's License #
Single	Student	SE69956571

Emergency Contact	Relationship to Patient	Phone Number
Darcy Logan	Mother	123-851-1061

RESPONSIBLE PARTY INFORMATION   SELF ☐

First Name	MI	Last Name		Date of Birth	Sex
Darcy		Logan		8/25/75	F

SSN	Home Phone	Work Phone		Cell
524-45-2460	123-851-1061			

Home Address	City	State	Zip
1412 Gina Dr	Anytown	AL	12345-1234

Employer		Relationship to Patient
		Mother

DENTAL INSURANCE INFORMATION

Primary Insurance Carrier	Phone Number
Delta Dental DMO	1-800-123-4545

Address	City	State	Zip
1255 Insurance Boulevard	Anytown	AL	12345-1234

Policy Holder Name (if different from patient)	Phone	Date of Birth	Sex
Darcy Logan	123-851-1061	8/25/75	F

Policy Number	Group Number	
VW3584926	452965F	

I hereby give lifetime authorization for payment of insurance benefits to be made directly to Walden-Martin Medical Group, and any assisting physicians, for services rendered. I understand that I am financially responsible for all charges whether or not they are covered by insurance. In the event of default, I agree to pay all costs of collection, and reasonable attorney's fees. I hereby authorize this healthcare provider to release all information necessary to secure the payment of benefits. I further agree that a photocopy of this agreement shall be as valid as the original.

Signature *Aaron T. Logan*	Date

Delta Dental   DMO

MEMBER NAME: Logan, Darcy

POLICY NUMBER: VW3584926
GROUP #: 452965F   EFFECTIVE DATE:
DEPENDENTS: Logan, Aaron   09/14/2015

CLAIMS/INQUIRIES: 1-800-123-4545

WALDEN-MARTIN
FAMILY MEDICAL CLINIC
1234 ANYSTREET | ANYTOWN, ANYSTATE 12345
PHONE 123-123-1234 | FAX 123-123-5678

JULIE WALDEN MD
JAMES MARTIN MD
DAVID KAHN MD
ANGELA PEREZ MD
PATRICK TAYLOR DDS
JEAN BURKE NP

PATIENT INFORMATION

First Name	MI	Last Name	Date of Birth	Sex
Ri		Liang	4/28/1948	M

SSN	Home Phone	Work Phone	Cell
177-16-3029	123-987-6565		

Home Address	City	State	Zip
101 Dalmation Dr	Anytown	AL	12345-1234

Marital Status	Employer	Driver's License #
Widowed	Retired	PW91590497

Emergency Contact	Relationship to Patient	Phone Number
Chen Liang		123-987-6565

RESPONSIBLE PARTY INFORMATION   SELF ☑

First Name	MI	Last Name	Date of Birth	Sex
Ri		Liang	4/28/1948	M

SSN	Home Phone	Work Phone	Cell
177-16-3029	123-987-6565		

Home Address	City	State	Zip
101 Dalmation Dr	Anytown	AL	12345-1234

Employer		Relationship to Patient
Retired		Self

INSURANCE INFORMATION

Primary Insurance Carrier	Phone Number
Medicare	1-800-123-3333

Address	City	State	Zip
1234 Insurance Road	Anytown	AL	12345-1234

Policy Holder Name (if different from patient)	Phone	Date of Birth	Sex

Policy Number	Group Number
486542027A	

Secondary Insurance Carrier	Phone Number

Address	City	State	Zip

Policy Holder Name (if different from patient)	Phone	Date of Birth	Sex

Policy Number	Group Number

I hereby give lifetime authorization for payment of insurance benefits to be made directly to Walden-Martin Medical Group, and any assisting physicians, for services rendered. I understand that I am financially responsible for all charges whether or not they are covered by insurance. In the event of default, I agree to pay all costs of collection, and reasonable attorney's fees. I hereby authorize this healthcare provider to release all information necessary to secure the payment of benefits. I further agree that a photocopy of this agreement shall be as valid as the original.

Signature *Ri Liang*	Date

MEDICARE   1234 Insurance Road

MEMBER NAME: Liang, Ri

POLICY #: 486542027A
EFFECTIVE DATE: 3/20/2015

Is entitled to:
HOSPITAL (PART A)
MEDICAL   (PART B)

CLAIMS/INQUIRIES: 1-800-123-3333

WALDEN-MARTIN
FAMILY MEDICAL CLINIC
1234 ANYSTREET | ANYTOWN, ANYSTATE 12345
PHONE 123-123-1234 | FAX 123-123-5678

JULIE WALDEN MD
JAMES MARTIN MD
DAVID KAHN MD
ANGELA PEREZ MD
PATRICK TAYLOR DDS
JEAN BURKE NP

PATIENT INFORMATION

First Name	MI	Last Name	Date of Birth	Sex
Kyle	R	Miller	12/27/1975	M

SSN	Home Phone	Work Phone	Cell
586-08-8591	123-853-7328		

Home Address	City	State	Zip
1325 Cherrywood St.	Anytown	AL	12345-1234

Marital Status	Employer	Driver's License #
Married	Anytown Steel Company	0530398625

Emergency Contact	Relationship to Patient	Phone Number
Sarah Miller	Wife	123-853-7328

RESPONSIBLE PARTY INFORMATION   SELF ☑

First Name	MI	Last Name	Date of Birth	Sex
Kyle	R	Miller	12/27/1975	M

SSN	Home Phone	Work Phone	Cell
586-08-8591	123-853-7328		

Home Address	City	State	Zip
1325 Cherrywood St.	Anytown	AL	12345-1234

Employer		Relationship to Patient
Anytown Steel Company		Self

INSURANCE INFORMATION

Primary Insurance Carrier	Phone Number
Southern Carpenters' Insurance Plan	1-800-123-6767

Address	City	State	Zip
1255 Insurance Street	Anytown	AL	12345-1234

Policy Holder Name (if different from patient)	Phone	Date of Birth	Sex

Policy Number	Group Number	
BS3630832	87462H	

Secondary Insurance Carrier	Phone Number

Address	City	State	Zip

Policy Holder Name (if different from patient)	Phone	Date of Birth	Sex

Policy Number	Group Number	

I hereby give lifetime authorization for payment of insurance benefits to be made directly to Walden-Martin Medical Group, and any assisting physicians, for services rendered. I understand that I am financially responsible for all charges whether or not they are covered by insurance. In the event of default, I agree to pay all costs of collection, and reasonable attorney's fees. I hereby authorize this healthcare provider to release all information necessary to secure the payment of benefits. I further agree that a photocopy of this agreement shall be as valid as the original.

Signature	Date
Kyle R. Miller	

SOUTHERN CARPENTER'S INSURANCE PLAN

MEMBER NAME: Miller, Kyle
POLICY NUMBER: BS3630832
GROUP #: 87462H
DEPENDENTS:

EFFECTIVE DATE:
09/14/2015

CO-PAY: $25
SPECIALIST CO-PAY: $35
XRAY/LAB BENEFIT: $250

DRUG CO-PAY
GENERIC: $10
NAME BRAND: $50

CLAIMS/INQUIRIES: 1-800-123-1234

WALDEN-MARTIN
FAMILY MEDICAL CLINIC
1234 ANYSTREET | ANYTOWN, ANYSTATE 12345
PHONE 123-123-1234 | FAX 123-123-5678

JULIE WALDEN MD
JAMES MARTIN MD
DAVID KAHN MD
ANGELA PEREZ MD
PATRICK TAYLOR DDS
JEAN BURKE NP

PATIENT INFORMATION

First Name	MI	Last Name	Date of Birth	Sex
Jill	M	Reinholt	2/16/1979	F

SSN	Home Phone	Work Phone	Cell
503-64-5774	123-989-2321		

Home Address	City	State	Zip
8771 Fairview Lane, Apt. 9	Anytown	AL	12345-1234

Marital Status	Employer	Driver's License #
Separated	Anytown Factory	ME27226410

Emergency Contact	Relationship to Patient	Phone Number
Katherine Drummon		123-409-5411

RESPONSIBLE PARTY INFORMATION   SELF ☑

First Name	MI	Last Name	Date of Birth	Sex
Jill	M	Reinholt	2/16/1979	F

SSN	Home Phone	Work Phone	Cell
503-64-5774	123-989-2321		

Home Address	City	State	Zip
8771 Fairview Lane, Apt. 9	Anytown	AL	12345-1234

Employer		Relationship to Patient
Anytown Factory		Self

INSURANCE INFORMATION

Primary Insurance Carrier	Phone Number
Seattle Casualty	1-800-123-9999

Address	City	State	Zip
1255 Insurance Lane	Anytown	AL	12345-1234

Policy Holder Name (if different from patient)	Phone	Date of Birth	Sex

Policy Number	Group Number
PF8431469	46291F

Secondary Insurance Carrier	Phone Number

Address	City	State	Zip

Policy Holder Name (if different from patient)	Phone	Date of Birth	Sex

Policy Number	Group Number

I hereby give lifetime authorization for payment of insurance benefits to be made directly to Walden-Martin Medical Group, and any assisting physicians, for services rendered. I understand that I am financially responsible for all charges whether or not they are covered by insurance. In the event of default, I agree to pay all costs of collection, and reasonable attorney's fees. I hereby authorize this healthcare provider to release all information necessary to secure the payment of benefits. I further agree that a photocopy of this agreement shall be as valid as the original.

Signature	Date
Jill Reinholt	

Seattle Casualty

MEMBER NAME: Reinholt, Jill

POLICY NUMBER: PF8431469
GROUP #: 46291F
DEPENDENTS:

EFFECTIVE DATE:
09/14/2015

CO-PAY: $25
SPECIALIST CO-PAY: $35
XRAY/LAB BENEFIT: $250

Care RX:
Rx Bin: 980146
Rx Group: 3515RX

CLAIMS/INQUIRIES: 1-800-123-9999

WALDEN-MARTIN
FAMILY MEDICAL CLINIC
1234 ANYSTREET | ANYTOWN, ANYSTATE 12345
PHONE 123-123-1234 | FAX 123-123-5678

JULIE WALDEN MD
JAMES MARTIN MD
DAVID KAHN MD
ANGELA PEREZ MD
PATRICK TAYLOR DDS
JEAN BURKE NP

PATIENT INFORMATION

First Name	MI	Last Name	Date of Birth	Sex
Christina		Brown	8/3/2001	F

SSN	Home Phone	Work Phone	Cell
503-18-1456	123-521-9686		

Home Address	City	State	Zip
89 Collins Way	Anytown	AL	12345-1234

Marital Status	Employer	Driver's License #
Single	Student	

Emergency Contact	Relationship to Patient	Phone Number
Mary Brown	Mother	123-251-9686

RESPONSIBLE PARTY INFORMATION   SELF ☐

First Name	MI	Last Name	Date of Birth	Sex
James		Brown	10/5/1975	M

SSN	Home Phone	Work Phone	Cell
869-50-5420	123-251-9686		

Home Address	City	State	Zip
89 Collins Way	Anytown	AL	12345-1234

Employer		Relationship to Patient
		Father

INSURANCE INFORMATION

Primary Insurance Carrier	Phone Number
Health First	1-800-123-7777

Address	City	State	Zip
1234 Insurance Boulevard	Anytown	AL	12345-1234

Policy Holder Name (if different from patient)	Phone	Date of Birth	Sex
James Brown	123-251-9686	10/5/1975	M

Policy Number	Group Number
NW9908272	16096T

Secondary Insurance Carrier	Phone Number

Address	City	State	Zip

Policy Holder Name (if different from patient)	Phone	Date of Birth	Sex

Policy Number	Group Number

I hereby give lifetime authorization for payment of insurance benefits to be made directly to Walden-Martin Medical Group, and any assisting physicians, for services rendered. I understand that I am financially responsible for all charges whether or not they are covered by insurance. In the event of default, I agree to pay all costs of collection, and reasonable attorney's fees. I hereby authorize this healthcare provider to release all information necessary to secure the payment of benefits. I further agree that a photocopy of this agreement shall be as valid as the original.

Signature *Christina Brown*	Date

HealthFirst

MEMBER NAME: Brown, James
POLICY NUMBER: NW9908272
GROUP #: 16096T
DEPENDENTS: Brown, Christina   **EFFECTIVE DATE:** 11/24/2015

Network Coinsurance:
In: 80% / 20%
Out: 60% / 40%

DRUG CO-PAY
GENERIC: $20
NAME BRAND: $50

CLAIMS/INQUIRIES: 1-800-123-7777

Front Office

WALDEN-MARTIN
FAMILY MEDICAL CLINIC
1234 ANYSTREET | ANYTOWN, ANYSTATE 12345
PHONE 123-123-1234 | FAX 123-123-5678

JULIE WALDEN MD
JAMES MARTIN MD
DAVID KAHN MD
ANGELA PEREZ MD
PATRICK TAYLOR DDS
JEAN BURKE NP

DENTAL

PATIENT INFORMATION

First Name	MI	Last Name	Date of Birth	Sex
Richard		Royer	3/18/23	M

SSN	Home Phone	Work Phone	Cell
414-24-1963	123-555-7008		

Home Address	City	State	Zip
1285 Ellery Avenue	Anytown	AL	12345-1234

Marital Status	Employer	Driver's License #
Widowed	Retired	PM22058420

Emergency Contact	Relationship to Patient	Phone Number
Richard Royer, Jr.	Son	123-555-7008

RESPONSIBLE PARTY INFORMATION   SELF ☑

First Name	MI	Last Name	Date of Birth	Sex
Richard		Royer	3/18/23	M

SSN	Home Phone	Work Phone	Cell
414-24-1963	123-555-7008		

Home Address	City	State	Zip
1285 Ellery Avenue	Anytown	AL	12345-1234

Employer		Relationship to Patient
Retired		Self

DENTAL INSURANCE INFORMATION

Primary Insurance Carrier	Phone Number
Medicare (Dental)	1-800-123-3333

Address	City	State	Zip
1234 Insurance Road	Anytown	AL	12345-1234

Policy Holder Name (if different from patient)	Phone	Date of Birth	Sex

Policy Number	Group Number	
293954644A		

I hereby give lifetime authorization for payment of insurance benefits to be made directly to Walden-Martin Medical Group, and any assisting physicians, for services rendered. I understand that I am financially responsible for all charges whether or not they are covered by insurance. In the event of default, I agree to pay all costs of collection, and reasonable attorney's fees. I hereby authorize this healthcare provider to release all information necessary to secure the payment of benefits. I further agree that a photocopy of this agreement shall be as valid as the original.

Signature	Date
Richard Royer	

MEDICARE Dental   1234 Insurance Road

MEMBER NAME: Royer, Richard

POLICY #: 293954644A
EFFECTIVE DATE: 3/20/2015

Is entitled to:
HOSPITAL   (PART A)
MEDICAL   (PART B)

CLAIMS/INQUIRIES: 1-800-123-3333

WALDEN-MARTIN
FAMILY MEDICAL CLINIC
1234 ANYSTREET | ANYTOWN, ANYSTATE 12345
PHONE 123-123-1234 | FAX 123-123-5678

JULIE WALDEN MD
JAMES MARTIN MD
DAVID KAHN MD
ANGELA PEREZ MD
PATRICK TAYLOR DDS
JEAN BURKE NP

PATIENT INFORMATION

First Name	MI	Last Name	Date of Birth	Sex
Margaret		Chan	8/26/1947	F

SSN	Home Phone	Work Phone	Cell
542-35-0077	123-851-9634		

Home Address	City	State	Zip
310 Cherry Blossom Dr	Anytown	AL	12345-1234

Marital Status	Employer	Driver's License #
Widowed	Retired	VW62061829

Emergency Contact	Relationship to Patient	Phone Number
Lilly Chan	Daughter	123-452-8543

RESPONSIBLE PARTY INFORMATION   SELF ☑

First Name	MI	Last Name	Date of Birth	Sex
Margaret		Chan	8/26/1947	F

SSN	Home Phone	Work Phone	Cell
542-35-0077	123-851-9634		

Home Address	City	State	Zip
310 Cherry Blossom Dr	Anytown	AL	12345-1234

Employer		Relationship to Patient
Retired		Self

INSURANCE INFORMATION

Primary Insurance Carrier	Phone Number
Medicare	1-800-123-3333

Address	City	State	Zip
1234 Insurance Road	Anytown	AL	12345-1234

Policy Holder Name (if different from patient)	Phone	Date of Birth	Sex

Policy Number	Group Number
510240661A	

Secondary Insurance Carrier	Phone Number

Address	City	State	Zip

Policy Holder Name (if different from patient)	Phone	Date of Birth	Sex

Policy Number	Group Number

I hereby give lifetime authorization for payment of insurance benefits to be made directly to Walden-Martin Medical Group, and any assisting physicians, for services rendered. I understand that I am financially responsible for all charges whether or not they are covered by insurance. In the event of default, I agree to pay all costs of collection, and reasonable attorney's fees. I hereby authorize this healthcare provider to release all information necessary to secure the payment of benefits. I further agree that a photocopy of this agreement shall be as valid as the original.

Signature *Margaret Chan*	Date

MEDICARE   1234 Insurance Road

MEMBER NAME: Chan, Margaret

POLICY #: 510240661A
EFFECTIVE DATE: 3/20/2015

Is entitled to:
HOSPITAL (PART A)
MEDICAL   (PART B)

CLAIMS/INQUIRIES: 1-800-123-3333

WALDEN-MARTIN
FAMILY MEDICAL CLINIC
1234 ANYSTREET | ANYTOWN, ANYSTATE 12345
PHONE 123-123-1234 | FAX 123-123-5678

JULIE WALDEN MD
JAMES MARTIN MD
DAVID KAHN MD
ANGELA PEREZ MD
PATRICK TAYLOR DDS
JEAN BURKE NP

DENTAL		

PATIENT INFORMATION

First Name	MI	Last Name	Date of Birth	Sex
Lillian	K	Chambers	1/10/76	F

SSN	Home Phone	Work Phone	Cell
157-89-3984	123-543-4747		

Home Address	City	State	Zip
1472 McGee St.	Anytown	AL	12345-1234

Marital Status	Employer	Driver's License #
Married	Unemployed	PV86132461

Emergency Contact	Relationship to Patient	Phone Number
Donald Chambers		123-543-4747

RESPONSIBLE PARTY INFORMATION   SELF ☑

First Name	MI	Last Name	Date of Birth	Sex
Lillian	K	Chambers	1/10/76	F

SSN	Home Phone	Work Phone	Cell
157-89-3984	123-543-4747		

Home Address	City	State	Zip
1472 McGee St.	Anytown	AL	12345-1234

Employer		Relationship to Patient
Unemployed		Self

DENTAL INSURANCE INFORMATION

Primary Insurance Carrier	Phone Number
Aetna PPO (Dental)	1-800-123-3434

Address	City	State	Zip
1234 Insurance Way	Anytown	AL	12345-1234

Policy Holder Name (if different from patient)	Phone	Date of Birth	Sex

Policy Number	Group Number
BY9365937	439563D

I hereby give lifetime authorization for payment of insurance benefits to be made directly to Walden-Martin Medical Group, and any assisting physicians, for services rendered. I understand that I am financially responsible for all charges whether or not they are covered by insurance. In the event of default, I agree to pay all costs of collection, and reasonable attorney's fees. I hereby authorize this healthcare provider to release all information necessary to secure the payment of benefits. I further agree that a photocopy of this agreement shall be as valid as the original.

Signature	Date
Lillian Chambers	

AETNA DENTAL PPO   1234 Insurance Way

MEMBER NAME: Lillian Chambers

POLICY #: BY9365937   **DEPENDENTS:**
GROUP #: 439563D   **EFFECTIVE DATE:**
02/01/2015

Member Services: 1-800-123-2222

Front Office

WALDEN-MARTIN
FAMILY MEDICAL CLINIC
1234 ANYSTREET | ANYTOWN, ANYSTATE 12345
PHONE 123-123-1234 | FAX 123-123-5678

JULIE WALDEN MD
JAMES MARTIN MD
DAVID KAHN MD
ANGELA PEREZ MD
PATRICK TAYLOR DDS
JEAN BURKE NP

PATIENT INFORMATION

First Name	MI	Last Name	Date of Birth	Sex
Ruby		Cleary	9/8/34	F

SSN	Home Phone	Work Phone	Cell
413-00-4111	123-338-8484		

Home Address	City	State	Zip
40 Cherry Orchard Rd.	Anytown	AL	12345-1234

Marital Status	Employer	Driver's License #
Widowed	Retired	LW79719735

Emergency Contact	Relationship to Patient	Phone Number
Robin Cleary	Daughter	123-338-8484

RESPONSIBLE PARTY INFORMATION   SELF ☑

First Name	MI	Last Name	Date of Birth	Sex
Ruby		Cleary	9/8/34	F

SSN	Home Phone	Work Phone	Cell
413-00-4111	123-338-8484		

Home Address	City	State	Zip
40 Cherry Orchard Rd.	Anytown	AL	12345-1234

Employer		Relationship to Patient
Retired		Self

INSURANCE INFORMATION

Primary Insurance Carrier	Phone Number
Medicare	1-800-123-3333

Address	City	State	Zip
1234 Insurance Road	Anytown	AL	12345-1234

Policy Holder Name (if different from patient)	Phone	Date of Birth	Sex

Policy Number	Group Number
SY7055985A	

Secondary Insurance Carrier	Phone Number

Address	City	State	Zip

Policy Holder Name (if different from patient)	Phone	Date of Birth	Sex

Policy Number	Group Number

I hereby give lifetime authorization for payment of insurance benefits to be made directly to Walden-Martin Medical Group, and any assisting physicians, for services rendered. I understand that I am financially responsible for all charges whether or not they are covered by insurance. In the event of default, I agree to pay all costs of collection, and reasonable attorney's fees. I hereby authorize this healthcare provider to release all information necessary to secure the payment of benefits. I further agree that a photocopy of this agreement shall be as valid as the original.

Signature	*Ruby Cleary*	Date	

MEDICARE   1234 Insurance Road

MEMBER NAME: Cleary, Ruby

POLICY #: SY7055985A
EFFECTIVE DATE: 01/01/2015

Is entitled to:
HOSPITAL (PART A)
MEDICAL   (PART B)

CLAIMS/INQUIRIES: 1-800-123-3333

WALDEN-MARTIN
FAMILY MEDICAL CLINIC
1234 ANYSTREET | ANYTOWN, ANYSTATE 12345
PHONE 123-123-1234 | FAX 123-123-5678

JULIE WALDEN MD
JAMES MARTIN MD
DAVID KAHN MD
ANGELA PEREZ MD
PATRICK TAYLOR DDS
JEAN BURKE NP

PATIENT INFORMATION

First Name	MI	Last Name	Date of Birth	Sex
Mary	L	Cohen	6/5/1966	F

SSN	Home Phone	Work Phone	Cell
440-92-1463	123-417-8744		

Home Address	City	State	Zip
1926 Ninth Ave.	Anytown	AL	12345-1234

Marital Status	Employer	Driver's License #
Divorced	Anytown Law Office	TN85962826

Emergency Contact	Relationship to Patient	Phone Number
Sara Cohen		123-854-9658

RESPONSIBLE PARTY INFORMATION   SELF ☑

First Name	MI	Last Name	Date of Birth	Sex
Mary	L	Cohen	6/5/1966	F

SSN	Home Phone	Work Phone	Cell
440-92-1463	123-417-8744		

Home Address	City	State	Zip
1926 Ninth Ave.	Anytown	AL	12345-1234

Employer		Relationship to Patient
Anytown Law Office		Self

INSURANCE INFORMATION

Primary Insurance Carrier	Phone Number
MetLife	1-800-123-4444

Address	City	State	Zip
1234 Insurance Avenue	Anytown	AL	12345-1234

Policy Holder Name (if different from patient)	Phone	Date of Birth	Sex

Policy Number	Group Number
LZ1124595	17267E

Secondary Insurance Carrier	Phone Number

Address	City	State	Zip

Policy Holder Name (if different from patient)	Phone	Date of Birth	Sex

Policy Number	Group Number

I hereby give lifetime authorization for payment of insurance benefits to be made directly to Walden-Martin Medical Group, and any assisting physicians, for services rendered. I understand that I am financially responsible for all charges whether or not they are covered by insurance. In the event of default, I agree to pay all costs of collection, and reasonable attorney's fees. I hereby authorize this healthcare provider to release all information necessary to secure the payment of benefits. I further agree that a photocopy of this agreement shall be as valid as the original.

Signature *Mary L. Cohen*	Date

MetLife   1234 Insurance Avenue

MEMBER NAME: Cohen, Mary

POLICY #: LZ1124595
GROUP #: 17267E   **EFFECTIVE DATE:**
                                        08/24/2015

CO-PAY: $25   DRUG CO-PAY
SPECIALIST CO-PAY: $35   GENERIC: $15
XRAY/LAB BENEFIT: $250   NAME BRAND: $30

CLAIMS/INQUIRIES: 1-800-123-4444

WALDEN-MARTIN
FAMILY MEDICAL CLINIC
1234 ANYSTREET | ANYTOWN, ANYSTATE 12345
PHONE 123-123-1234 | FAX 123-123-5678

JULIE WALDEN MD
JAMES MARTIN MD
DAVID KAHN MD
ANGELA PEREZ MD
PATRICK TAYLOR DDS
JEAN BURKE NP

DENTAL

PATIENT INFORMATION

First Name	MI	Last Name	Date of Birth	Sex
Emilia	C	Garcia	1/24/2008	F

SSN	Home Phone	Work Phone	Cell
947-84-5107	123-221-1212		

Home Address	City	State	Zip
6252 Seacrest Dr., Apt. 121	Anytown	AL	12345-1234

Marital Status	Employer	Driver's License #
Single	None	

Emergency Contact	Relationship to Patient	Phone Number
Consuelo Garcia	Mother	123-221-1212

RESPONSIBLE PARTY INFORMATION   SELF ☐

First Name	MI	Last Name	Date of Birth	Sex
Consuelo		Garcia	6/30/1979	F

SSN	Home Phone	Work Phone	Cell
947-84-5107	123-221-1212		

Home Address	City	State	Zip
6252 Seacrest Dr., Apt. 121	Anytown	AL	12345-1234

Employer	Relationship to Patient
	Mother

DENTAL INSURANCE INFORMATION

Primary Insurance Carrier	Phone Number
Aetna PPO (Dental)	1-800-123-3434

Address	City	State	Zip
1234 Insurance Way	Anytown	AL	12345-1234

Policy Holder Name (if different from patient)	Phone	Date of Birth	Sex
Consuelo Garcia	123-221-1212	6/30/1979	F

Policy Number	Group Number
UN2784681	548396B

I hereby give lifetime authorization for payment of insurance benefits to be made directly to Walden-Martin Medical Group, and any assisting physicians, for services rendered. I understand that I am financially responsible for all charges whether or not they are covered by insurance. In the event of default, I agree to pay all costs of collection, and reasonable attorney's fees. I hereby authorize this healthcare provider to release all information necessary to secure the payment of benefits. I further agree that a photocopy of this agreement shall be as valid as the original.

Signature	Date
Emilia Garcia	

AETNA DENTAL PPO   1234 Insurance Way

MEMBER NAME: Consuelo Garcia

POLICY #: UN2784681
GROUP #: 548396B

DEPENDENTS: Emilia Garcia
EFFECTIVE DATE: 02/20/2015

Member Services: 1-800-123-2222

 Now complete the Review Questions for this unit on your Evolve site.

Unit 3 | Claim Entry

Completing superbills and submitting claims are steps at the end of the patient workflow and are necessary for keeping the business end of a practice running smoothly. After a patient is seen in the office and the encounter is documented by the provider, it is important for that data to be translated into the correct coding for the practice to be paid for services rendered. Without an accurate and efficient billing process, a practice has little chance for success.

Generating a superbill (also called an encounter form, charge slip, routing slip, fee slip, or check-out form) entails assigning procedure and diagnosis codes to a patient visit and determining costs associated with those procedures. A superbill is tied to a particular encounter and cannot be generated unless an encounter is already entered in the system. The person tasked with the coding of the superbill will use the information from the encounter to determine the correct procedure and diagnosis codes for a visit. A patient could have one or more procedure and/or diagnosis code applied to any one visit, and there are more codes available for the average person to ever know by heart.

The TruCode encoder tool (Figure 3-1) in SimChart for the Medical Office contains a set of both procedure and diagnosis codes with explanations of each. This tool can be used for reference at any point in the process, or used to populate codes into specific fields while completing the superbill. After the codes are determined for a specific procedure, the practice's fee schedule (Figure 3-2) can be accessed to determine the associated costs. When all of the codes and costs have been determined, it is time to submit the claim.

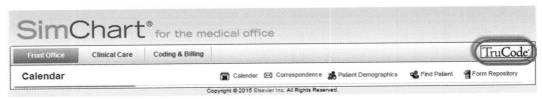

Figure 3-1 TruCode encoder tool.

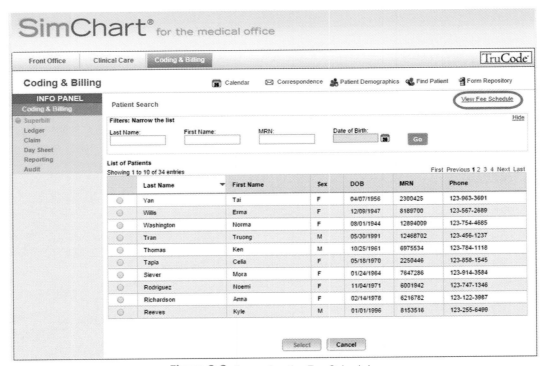

Figure 3-2 Accessing the Fee Schedule.

Claims are forms submitted to insurance carriers for processing and reimbursement of services. It is very important that claims are submitted correctly to avoid rejections from carriers. Claims can be submitted in either paper or electronic format. With medical claims the paper format is the CMS-1500 and the electronic format is the HIPAA 5010. In the dental field the J430D is used for claims submission. A mock form has been developed for SimChart for the Medical Office to model the form for dental reimbursement. Medical and dental insurance companies ask for much of the same information from health professionals, but there are some minor differences between the two, the largest being that although dental claims require procedure codes, at this time diagnosis codes are not required.

Like superbills, claims are also accessed through the Coding & Billing module of the system (Figure 3-3), but it is only possible to submit a claim if a superbill for a patient encounter has already been completed.

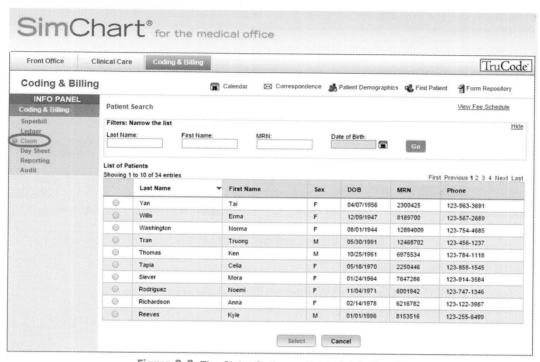

Figure 3-3 The Claim Option on the Left Info Panel.

Submitting a Superbill

Norma Washington has been seeing Dr. Martin for degenerative joint disease in her right knee. She had a follow up visit on 08/14/2015 to discuss her medications. Dr. Martin has indicated that this visit had an expanded problem-focused history, an expanded problem-focused examination, and medical decision making of low complexity. The patient made no payment at the time of the visit. Use the TruCode encoder and Fee Schedule to complete and submit a superbill for Ms. Washington.

Measurable Steps

1. Click the Find Patient icon (Figure 3-4).

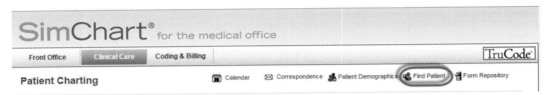

Figure 3-4 The Find Patient Icon.

2. Using the Patient Search field, search for Norma Washington's patient record.
3. Select the radio button for Norma Washington and click the select button.
4. Confirm the autopopulated details in the Patient Header.
5. After reviewing the encounter, click the Superbill link below the Patient Header (Figure 3-5).

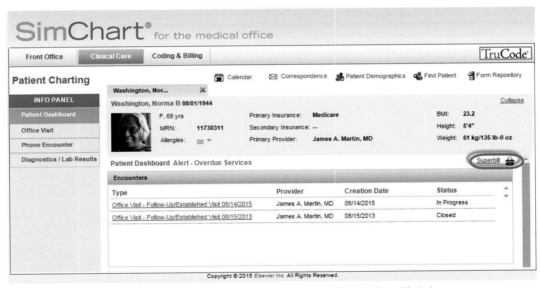

Figure 3-5 Accessing the Superbill from the Clinical Care Module.

6. Select the correct encounter from the Encounters Not Coded table and confirm the autopopulated details.
7. Select the ICD-10 radio button.
8. In the Rank 1 row of the Diagnoses box, place the cursor in the text field to access the encoder (Figure 3-6).

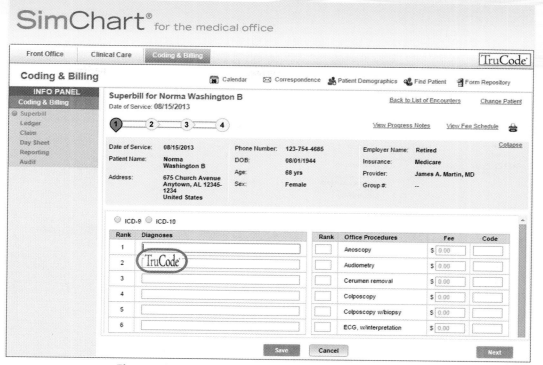

Figure 3-6 Accessing the Encoder from the Diagnosis Box.

9. Enter "degenerative joint disease" in the Search field, select Diagnosis ICD-10-CM from the dropdown menu, and click the Search button.

10. Select "Osteoarthritis" in the Book: ICD-10-CM Diagnosis box and search for the code for osteoarthritis in the knee and select it.

11. Review M17.9 to ensure that this is the most specific code available. Select this code and it will autopopulate in the Rank 1 row of the Diagnoses box (Figure 3-7).

12. In the office visit section, enter "1" in the Rank column next to Expanded problem-focused visit to tie the osteoarthritis diagnosis to this procedure.

13. Place the cursor in the Est. column of that row to access the TruCode encoder to look up the code for this type of encounter.

14. Enter "Expanded problem focused" in the search field, select CPT Tabular from the dropdown menu, and click the Search button.

15. Select the correct CPT code and it will autopopulate in the superbill.

16. Open the Fee Schedule using the link at the top and use the code you discovered in step 15 to determine the fee of Norma Washington's visit and document this amount in the Fee column next to the office visit.

17. Click the Save button.

18. Click the Next button three times to advance to the fourth page of the superbill.

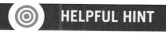 **HELPFUL HINT**

Because Norma Washington did not make any payments on her account at the time of visit, the Balance Due will match the total charges of the visit. Had she made a copayment, that amount would have been subtracted from today's charges, leaving a smaller balance due.

19. Select the Same Name as Patient checkbox below the Insured's Name field to indicate that Norma Washington is the insured patient for the visit. Her name should populate in the appropriate fields.

20. Select the Same Address as Patient checkbox below the Insured's Address field. Norma Washington's address should populate in the appropriate field.

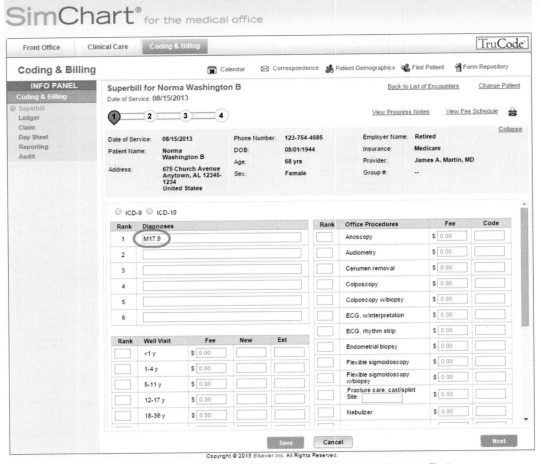

Figure 3-7 The Diagnosis Code Autopopulating from the Encoder Tool.

21. Select the Self radio button in the Patient Relationship to Insured field.
22. Select the Married radio button in the Patient Status field.
23. Select the No radio button to indicate that there are no other health benefits.
24. Select the No radio buttons to indicate that the patient condition is not related to employment or an accident.
25. Click the Save button.
26. Select the "I am ready to submit the Superbill" checkbox at the bottom of the screen.
27. Select the Yes radio button to indicate that the signature is on file.
28. Document the date in the Date field.
29. Click the Submit Superbill button. A confirmation message will appear (Figure 3-8).

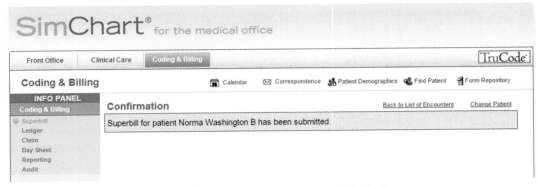

Figure 3-8 Confirmation of Superbill Submission.

Activity

Complete superbills in SimChart for the Medical Office using the superbills printed on the following pages.

WALDEN-MARTIN
FAMILY MEDICAL CLINIC
1234 ANYSTREET | ANYTOWN, ANYSTATE 12345
PHONE 123-123-1234 | FAX 123-123-5678

JULIE WALDEN MD
JAMES MARTIN MD
DAVID KAHN MD
ANGELA PEREZ MD
PATRICK TAYLOR DDS
JEAN BURKE NP

Patient Name: Butler, Janine
DOS: 11/18/2015
Diagnoses 1): J02.0
2):
3):
4):

SERVICE	CODE New	Est.	PRICE	SERVICE	CODE	PRICE	SERVICE	CODE	PRICE
OFFICE VISIT	New	Est.		MEDICATIONS CONT'D			LABORATORY CONT'D		
MINIMAL OFFICE VISIT (OV)	99201	99211		B-12, UP TO 1,000MCG	J3420		STREP, RAPID	87880	
PROBLEM FOCUSED OV	99202	99212		EPINEPHINE, UP TO 1ML	J0170		STREP CULTURE	87081	38.00
EXPANDED OV	99203	99213	43.00	KENALOG, 10MG	J3301		TB	87116	
DETAILED OV	99204	99214		LIDCAINE, 10MG	J2001		UA, COMPLETE, NON-AUTOMATED, MICRO	81000	
COMPHREHENSIVE OV	99205	99215		PROGESTERONE, 150MG	J1055		UA, W/O MICRO NON-AUTOMATED	81002	
WELLNESS VISIT	New	Est.		RECEPHIN, 250MG	J0696		UA, W/ MICRO, NON-AUTOMATED	81001	
WELL VISIT < 1 Y	99381	99391		TESTOSTERONE, 200MG	J1080		URINE COLONY COUNT	87086	
WELL VISIT 1-4 Y	99382	99392		TIGAN, UP TO 200MG	J3250		WET MOUNT/KOH	87210	
WELL VISIT 5-11 Y	99383	99393		TORADOL, 15MG	J1885		INPATIENT/OUTPATIENT PROCEDURES		
WELL VISIT 12-17 Y	99384	99394		NORMAL SALINE, 1000CC	J7030		UPPER GI ENDOSCOPY	43235	
WELL VISIT 18-39 Y	99385	99395		PHENERGAN, UP TO 50MG	J2550		UPPER GI ENDOSCOPY W/ BIOPSY	43239	
WELL VISIT 40-64 Y	99386	99396		IMMUNIZATIONS & INJECTIONS			UPPER GI ENDOSCOPY W/ GUIDE WIRE	43248	
WELL VISIT 65 Y+	99387	99397		ALLERGEN, ONE	95115		UPPER GI ENDOSCOPY W/ BALLOON	43249	
PREVENTATIVE SERVICES				ALLERGEN, MULTIPLE	95117		COLONOSCOPY	45378	
PAP	Q0091			IMM ADMIN, ONE	90471		COLONOSCOPY W/ BIOPSY	45380	
PELVIC & BREAST	G0101			IMM ADMIN, EACH ADD'L	90472		COLONOSCOPY W/ BIOPSY REMOVAL	45384	
PROSTATE/PSA	G0103			IMM ADMIN, INTRANASAL, ONE	90473		COLONOSCOPY W/ SNARE REMOVAL	45385	
TOBACCO COUNSELING/3-10MIN	99406			IMM ADMIN, INTRANASAL, EACH ADD'L	90475		SKIN PROCEDURES		
TOBACCO COUNSELING/>10MIN	99407			INJECTION, JOINT, SMALL	206--		BURN CARE, INITIAL	16000	
WELCOME TO MEDICARE EXAM	G0366			INJECTION, THER/PROPH/DIAG	90772		FROEIGN BODY, SKIN, SIMPLE	10120	
ECG W/ WELCOME TO MEDICARE EXAM	G0366			INJECTION, TRIGGER POINT	20552		FOREIGN BODY, SKIN, COMPLEX	12121	
FLEXIBLE SIGMOIDOSCOPY	G0104			VACCINES			I&D, ABSCESS	10060	
HEMOCCULT, GUAIAC	G0107			DT, <7 Y	90702		I&D, HEMATOMA/SEROMA	10140	
FLU ADMINISTRATION	G0008			DTP	90701		LCERATION REPAIR, SIMPLE	120--	
PENUMONIA ADMINISTRATION	G0009			DTAP, <7 Y	90700		LACERATION REPAIR, LAYERED	120--	
CONSULTATION/PRE-OP CLEARANCE				FLU, 6-35 MONTHS	90657		LESION, BIOPSY, ONE	11100	
EXPANDED PROBLEM FOCUSED	99242			FLU, 3Y+	90658		LESION, BIOPSY, EACH ADD'L	11101	
DETAILED	99243			HEP A, PED/ADOL, 2 DOSE	90633		LESION, DEST., BENIGN 1-14	17110	
COMPREHENSIVE/MOD COMPLEXITY	99244			HEP A, ADULT	90632		LESION DEST., PRE-MAL., SINGLE	17000	
COMPREHENSIVE/HIGH COMPLEXITY	99245			HEP B, PED/ADOL, 3 DOSE	90744		LESION DEST., PRE-MAL., EACH ADD'L	17003	
OTHER SERVICES				HEP B, ADULT	90746		LESION, EXCISION BENIGN	114--	
AFTER POSTED HOURS	99050			HEP B-HIB	90748		LESION, EXCISION, MALIGNANT	116--	
EVENING/WEEKEND APPT.	99051			HIB, 4 DOSE	90645		LESION, PARING/CUTTING, ONE	11055	
HOME HEALTH CERTIFICATION	G0180			HPV	90649		LESION PARING/CUTTING 2-4	11056	
HOME HEALTH RECERTIFICATION	G0179			IPV	90713		LESION, SHAVE	113--	
POST-OP FOLLOW UP	99024			MMR	90707		NAIL REMOVAL, PARTIAL	11730	
PROLONGED/30-74MIN	99354			PNEUMONIA, >2 Y	90732		NAIL REMOVAL, W/ MATRIX	11750	
SPECIAL REPORTS/FORMS	99080			PNEUMONIA CONJUGATE, <5Y	90669		SKIN TA, 1-15	11200	
DISABILITY/WORKERS COMP	99455			TD, > 7Y	90718		DENTAL (For practice purposes only)		
SPECIMIN HANDLING	99000			VARICELLA	90716		PERIODIC ORAL EVALUATION	DE0100	
OFFICE PROCEDURES				LABORATORY			COMPREHENSIVE EVALUATION	DE0150	
ANOSCOPY	46600			VENIPUNCTURE	36415		INTRAORAL, PERIAPICAL – 1ST FILM	DE0200	
AUDIOMETRY	92551			BLOOD GLUCOSE, MONITORING DEVICE	82962		INTRAORAL, PERIAPICAL–EACH ADD'L FILM	DE0250	
CERUMEN REMOVAL	69210			BLOOD GLUCOSE, VISUAL DIPSTICK	82948		BITEWING	DE026-	
COLPOSCOPY	54752			CBC, W/ AUTO DIFFERENTIAL	85025		PROPHYLAXIS - ADULT	DE1000	
COLPOSCOPY W/ BIOPSY	57455			CBC, W/O AUTO DIFFRENTIAL	85027		PROPHYLAXIS - CHILD	DE2000	
ECG W/ INTERPRETATION	93000			CHOLESTEROL	82465		PERIODONTAL MAINT.	DE5000	
ECG, RHYTHM STRIP	93040			HEMOOCULT, GUAIAC	82272		RESTORATIVE (ANTERIOR)	DE250-	
ENDOMETRIAL BIOPSY	58100			HEMOCCULT, IMMUNOASSAY	82274		RESTORATIVE (POSTERIOR)	DE260-	
FLEXIBLE SIGMOIDOSCOPY	45330			HEMOGLOBIN A1C	83036		FUSE CROWN-PORC	DE2700	
FLEXIBLE SIGMOIDOSCOPY W/ BIOPSY	45331			LIPID PANEL	80061		RE-CEMENT CROWN	DE2900	
FRACTURE CARE, CAST/SPLINT	29---			LIVER PANEL	80076		CORE BUILD UP INC. PINS	DE3000	
NEBULIZER	94640			KHO PREP (SKIN, HAIR, NAILS)	87220		CORE BUILD UP, PREFAB POST	DE3250	
NEBULIZER DEMO	94664			METABOLIC PANEL, BASIC	80048		LABIAL VENEER	DE3500	
SPIROMETRY	94010			METABOLIC PANEL, COMPHREHENSIVE	80053		CROWN - PORCELAIN FUSED TO GOLD	DE6000	
SPIROMETRY, PRE AND POST	94060			MONONUCLEOSIS	86663		CROWN LENGTHENING	DE4000	
TYMPANOMETRY	92567			PREGNANCY, BLOOD	84702		SURGICAL EXTRACTION	DE7000	
VASECTOMY	55250			PREGNANCY, URINE	81025		IMPACTED EXTRACTION	DE7250	
MEDICATIONS				RENAL PANEL	80069		LTD. ORTHO TREATMENT, ADULT	DE8000	
AMPICILIN, UP TO 500MG	J0290			SEDIMENTATION RATE	85652		ANALGESIA, NITROUS OXIDE	DE9000	

TODAY'S FEE		81.00
AMOUNT RECEIVED		0.00
BALANCE		81.00

WALDEN-MARTIN
FAMILY MEDICAL CLINIC
1234 ANYSTREET | ANYTOWN, ANYSTATE 12345
PHONE 123-123-1234 | FAX 123-123-5678

JULIE WALDEN MD
JAMES MARTIN MD
DAVID KAHN MD
ANGELA PEREZ MD
PATRICK TAYLOR DDS
JEAN BURKE NP

Patient Name: Jackson, Aaron
DOS: 11/20/2015
Diagnoses 1): D64.9
2):
3):
4):

SERVICE	CODE		PRICE	SERVICE	CODE	PRICE	SERVICE	CODE	PRICE
OFFICE VISIT	New	Est.		MEDICATIONS CONT'D			LABORATORY CONT'D		
MINIMAL OFFICE VISIT (OV)	99201	99211		B-12, UP TO 1,000MCG	J3420		STREP, RAPID	87880	
PROBLEM FOCUSED OV	99202	99212		EPINEPHINE, UP TO 1ML	J0170		STREP CULTURE	87081	
EXPANDED OV	99203	99213	43.00	KENALOG, 10MG	J3301		TB	87116	
DETAILED OV	99204	99214		LIDCAINE, 10MG	J2001		UA, COMPLETE, NON-AUTOMATED, MICRO	81000	
COMPHREHENSIVE OV	99205	99215		PROGESTERONE, 150MG	J1055		UA, W/O MICRO NON-AUTOMATED	81002	
WELLNESS VISIT	New	Est.		RECEPHIN, 250MG	J0696		UA, W/ MICRO, NON-AUTOMATED	81001	
WELL VISIT < 1 Y	99381	99391		TESTOSTERONE, 200MG	J1080		URINE COLONY COUNT	87086	
WELL VISIT 1-4 Y	99382	99392		TIGAN, UP TO 200MG	J3250		WET MOUNT/KOH	87210	
WELL VISIT 5-11 Y	99383	99393		TORADOL, 15MG	J1885		INPATIENT/OUTPATIENT PROCEDURES		
WELL VISIT 12-17 Y	99384	99394		NORMAL SALINE, 1000CC	J7030		UPPER GI ENDOSCOPY	43235	
WELL VISIT 18-39 Y	99385	99395		PHENERGAN, UP TO 50MG	J2550		UPPER GI ENDOSCOPY W/ BIOPSY	43239	
WELL VISIT 40-64 Y	99386	99396		IMMUNIZATIONS & INJECTIONS			UPPER GI ENDOSCOPY W/ GUIDE WIRE	43248	
WELL VISIT 65 Y+	99387	99397		ALLERGEN, ONE	95115		UPPER GI ENDOSCOPY W/ BALLOON	43249	
PREVENTATIVE SERVICES				ALLERGEN, MULTIPLE	95117		COLONOSCOPY	45378	
PAP	Q0091			IMM ADMIN, ONE	90471		COLONOSCOPY W/ BIOPSY	45380	
PELVIC & BREAST	G0101			IMM ADMIN, EACH ADD'L	90472		COLONOSCOPY W/ BIOPSY REMOVAL	45384	
PROSTATE/PSA	G0103			IMM ADMIN, INTRANASAL, ONE	90473		COLONOSCOPY W/ SNARE REMOVAL	45385	
TOBACCO COUNSELING/3-10MIN	99406			IMM ADMIN, INTRANASAL, EACH ADD'L	90475		SKIN PROCEDURES		
TOBACCO COUNSELING/>10MIN	99407			INJECTION, JOINT, SMALL	206--		BURN CARE, INITIAL	16000	
WELCOME TO MEDICARE EXAM	G0366			INJECTION, THER/PROPH/DIAG	90772		FROEIGN BODY, SKIN, SIMPLE	10120	
ECG W/ WELCOME TO MEDICARE EXAM	G0366			INJECTION, TRIGGER POINT	20552		FOREIGN BODY, SKIN, COMPLEX	12121	
FLEXIBLE SIGMOIDOSCOPY	G0104			VACCINES			I&D, ABSCESS	10060	
HEMOCCULT, GUAIAC	G0107			DT, <7 Y	90702		I&D, HEMATOMA/SEROMA	10140	
FLU ADMINISTRATION	G0008			DTP	90701		LCERATION REPAIR, SIMPLE	120--	
PENUMONIA ADMINISTRATION	G0009			DTAP, <7 Y	90700		LACERATION REPAIR, LAYERED	120--	
CONSULTATION/PRE-OP CLEARANCE				FLU, 6-35 MONTHS	90657		LESION, BIOPSY, ONE	11100	
EXPANDED PROBLEM FOCUSED	99242			FLU, 3Y+	90658		LESION, BIOPSY, EACH ADD'L	11101	
DETAILED	99243			HEP A, PED/ADOL, 2 DOSE	90633		LESION, DEST., BENIGN 1-14	17110	
COMPREHENSIVE/MOD COMPLEXITY	99244			HEP A, ADULT	90632		LESION DEST., PRE-MAL., SINGLE	17000	
COMPREHENSIVE/HIGH COMPLEXITY	99245			HEP B, PED/ADOL, 3 DOSE	90744		LESION DEST., PRE-MAL., EACH ADD'L	17003	
OTHER SERVICES				HEP B, ADULT	90746		LESION, EXCISION BENIGN	114--	
AFTER POSTED HOURS	99050			HEP B-HIB	90748		LESION, EXCISION, MALIGNANT	116--	
EVENING/WEEKEND APPT.	99051			HIB, 4 DOSE	90645		LESION, PARING/CUTTING, ONE	11055	
HOME HEALTH CERTIFICATION	G0180			HPV	90649		LESION PARING/CUTTING 2-4	11056	
HOME HEALTH RECERTIFICATION	G0179			IPV	90713		LESION, SHAVE	113--	
POST-OP FOLLOW UP	99024			MMR	90707		NAIL REMOVAL, PARTIAL	11730	
PROLONGED/30-74MIN	99354			PNEUMONIA, >2 Y	90732		NAIL REMOVAL, W/ MATRIX	11750	
SPECIAL REPORTS/FORMS	99080			PNEUMONIA CONJUGATE, <5Y	90669		SKIN TA, 1-15	11200	
DISABILITY/WORKERS COMP	99455			TD, > 7Y	90718		DENTAL (For practice purposes only)		
SPECIMIN HANDLING	99000			VARICELLA	90716		PERIODIC ORAL EVALUATION	DE0100	
OFFICE PROCEDURES				LABORATORY			COMPREHENSIVE EVALUATION	DE0150	
ANOSCOPY	46600			VENIPUNCTURE	36415		INTRAORAL, PERIAPICAL – 1ST FILM	DE0200	
AUDIOMETRY	92551			BLOOD GLUCOSE, MONITORING DEVICE	82962		INTRAORAL, PERIAPICAL–EACH ADD'L FILM	DE0250	
CERUMEN REMOVAL	69210			BLOOD GLUCOSE, VISUAL DIPSTICK	82948		BITEWING	DE026-	
COLPOSCOPY	54752			CBC, W/ AUTO DIFFERENTIAL	85025		PROPHYLAXIS - ADULT	DE1000	
COLPOSCOPY W/ BIOPSY	57455			CBC, W/O AUTO DIFFRENTIAL	85027		PROPHYLAXIS - CHILD	DE2000	
ECG W/ INTERPRETATION	93000			CHOLESTEROL	82465		PERIODONTAL MAINT.	DE5000	
ECG, RHYTHM STRIP	93040			HEMOOCULT, GUAIAC	82272		RESTORATIVE (ANTERIOR)	DE250-	
ENDOMETRIAL BIOPSY	58100			HEMOCCULT, IMMUNOASSAY	82274		RESTORATIVE (POSTERIOR)	DE260-	
FLEXIBLE SIGMOIDOSCOPY	45330			HEMOGLOBIN A1C	83036		FUSE CROWN-PORC	DE2700	
FLEXIBLE SIGMOIDOSCOPY W/ BIOPSY	45331			LIPID PANEL	80061		RE-CEMENT CROWN	DE2900	
FRACTURE CARE, CAST/SPLINT	29---			LIVER PANEL	80076		CORE BUILD UP INC. PINS	DE3000	
NEBULIZER	94640			KHO PREP (SKIN, HAIR, NAILS)	87220		CORE BUILD UP, PREFAB POST	DE3250	
NEBULIZER DEMO	94664			METABOLIC PANEL, BASIC	80048		LABIAL VENEER	DE3500	
SPIROMETRY	94010			METABOLIC PANEL, COMPHREHENSIVE	80053		CROWN - PORCELAIN FUSED TO GOLD	DE6000	
SPIROMETRY, PRE AND POST	94060			MONONUCLEOSIS	86663		CROWN LENGTHENING	DE4000	
TYMPANOMETRY	92567			PREGNANCY, BLOOD	84702		SURGICAL EXTRACTION	DE7000	
VASECTOMY	55250			PREGNANCY, URINE	81025		IMPACTED EXTRACTION	DE7250	
MEDICATIONS				RENAL PANEL	80069		LTD. ORTHO TREATMENT, ADULT	DE8000	
AMPICILIN, UP TO 500MG	J0290			SEDIMENTATION RATE	85652		ANALGESIA, NITROUS OXIDE	DE9000	

TODAY'S FEE		43.00
AMOUNT RECEIVED		25.00
BALANCE		18.00

Claim Entry

WALDEN-MARTIN
FAMILY MEDICAL CLINIC
1234 ANYSTREET | ANYTOWN, ANYSTATE 12345
PHONE 123-123-1234 | FAX 123-123-5678

JULIE WALDEN MD
JAMES MARTIN MD
DAVID KAHN MD
ANGELA PEREZ MD
PATRICK TAYLOR DDS
JEAN BURKE NP

Patient Name: Yan, Tai
DOS: 11/13/2015
Diagnoses 1): Z00.129
2):
3):
4):

SERVICE	CODE		PRICE	SERVICE	CODE	PRICE	SERVICE	CODE	PRICE
OFFICE VISIT	New	Est.		MEDICATIONS CONT'D			LABORATORY CONT'D		
MINIMAL OFFICE VISIT (OV)	99201	99211		B-12, UP TO 1,000MCG	J3420		STREP, RAPID	87880	
PROBLEM FOCUSED OV	99202	99212		EPINEPHINE, UP TO 1ML	J0170		STREP CULTURE	87081	
EXPANDED OV	99203	99213		KENALOG, 10MG	J3301		TB	87116	
DETAILED OV	99204	99214		LIDCAINE, 10MG	J2001		UA, COMPLETE, NON-AUTOMATED, MICRO	81000	
COMPHREHENSIVE OV	99205	99215		PROGESTERONE, 150MG	J1055		UA, W/O MICRO NON-AUTOMATED	81002	
WELLNESS VISIT	New	Est.		RECEPHIN, 250MG	J0696		UA, W/ MICRO, NON-AUTOMATED	81001	
WELL VISIT < 1 Y	99381	99391		TESTOSTERONE, 200MG	J1080		URINE COLONY COUNT	87086	
WELL VISIT 1-4 Y	99382	99392		TIGAN, UP TO 200MG	J3250		WET MOUNT/KOH	87210	
WELL VISIT 5-11 Y	99383	99393		TORADOL, 15MG	J1885		INPATIENT/OUTPATIENT PROCEDURES		
WELL VISIT 12-17 Y	99384	99394		NORMAL SALINE, 1000CC	J7030		UPPER GI ENDOSCOPY	43235	
WELL VISIT 18-39 Y	99385	99395		PHENERGAN, UP TO 50MG	J2550		UPPER GI ENDOSCOPY W/ BIOPSY	43239	
WELL VISIT 40-64 Y	99386	99396	70.00	IMMUNIZATIONS & INJECTIONS			UPPER GI ENDOSCOPY W/ GUIDE WIRE	43248	
WELL VISIT 65 Y+	99387	99397		ALLERGEN, ONE	95115		UPPER GI ENDOSCOPY W/ BALLOON	43249	
PREVENTATIVE SERVICES				ALLERGEN, MULTIPLE	95117		COLONOSCOPY	45378	
PAP	Q0091			IMM ADMIN, ONE	90471		COLONOSCOPY W/ BIOPSY	45380	
PELVIC & BREAST	G0101			IMM ADMIN, EACH ADD'L	90472		COLONOSCOPY W/ BIOPSY REMOVAL	45384	
PROSTATE/PSA	G0103			IMM ADMIN, INTRANASAL, ONE	90473		COLONOSCOPY W/ SNARE REMOVAL	45385	
TOBACCO COUNSELING/3-10MIN	99406			IMM ADMIN, INTRANASAL, EACH ADD'L	90475		SKIN PROCEDURES		
TOBACCO COUNSELING/>10MIN	99407			INJECTION, JOINT, SMALL	206--		BURN CARE, INITIAL	16000	
WELCOME TO MEDICARE EXAM	G0366			INJECTION, THER/PROPH/DIAG	90772		FROEIGN BODY, SKIN, SIMPLE	10120	
ECG W/ WELCOME TO MEDICARE EXAM	G0366			INJECTION, TRIGGER POINT	20552		FOREIGN BODY, SKIN, COMPLEX	12121	
FLEXIBLE SIGMOIDOSCOPY	G0104			VACCINES			I&D, ABSCESS	10060	
HEMOCCULT, GUAIAC	G0107			DT, <7 Y	90702		I&D, HEMATOMA/SEROMA	10140	
FLU ADMINISTRATION	G0008			DTP	90701		LCERATION REPAIR, SIMPLE	120--	
PENUMONIA ADMINISTRATION	G0009			DTAP, <7 Y	90700		LACERATION REPAIR, LAYERED	120--	
CONSULTATION/PRE-OP CLEARANCE				FLU, 6-35 MONTHS	90657		LESION, BIOPSY, ONE	11100	
EXPANDED PROBLEM FOCUSED	99242			FLU, 3Y+	90658		LESION, BIOPSY, EACH ADD'L	11101	
DETAILED	99243			HEP A, PED/ADOL, 2 DOSE	90633		LESION, DEST., BENIGN 1-14	17110	
COMPREHENSIVE/MOD COMPLEXITY	99244			HEP A, ADULT	90632		LESION DEST., PRE-MAL., SINGLE	17000	
COMPREHENSIVE/HIGH COMPLEXITY	99245			HEP B, PED/ADOL, 3 DOSE	90744		LESION DEST., PRE-MAL., EACH ADD'L	17003	
OTHER SERVICES				HEP B, ADULT	90746		LESION, EXCISION BENIGN	114--	
AFTER POSTED HOURS	99050			HEP B-HIB	90748		LESION, EXCISION, MALIGNANT	116--	
EVENING/WEEKEND APPT.	99051			HIB, 4 DOSE	90645		LESION, PARING/CUTTING, ONE	11055	
HOME HEALTH CERTIFICATION	G0180			HPV	90649		LESION PARING/CUTTING 2-4	11056	
HOME HEALTH RECERTIFICATION	G0179			IPV	90713		LESION, SHAVE	113--	
POST-OP FOLLOW UP	99024			MMR	90707		NAIL REMOVAL, PARTIAL	11730	
PROLONGED/30-74MIN	99354			PNEUMONIA, >2 Y	90732		NAIL REMOVAL, W/ MATRIX	11750	
SPECIAL REPORTS/FORMS	99080			PNEUMONIA CONJUGATE, <5Y	90669		SKIN TA, 1-15	11200	
DISABILITY/WORKERS COMP	99455			TD, > 7Y	90718		DENTAL (For practice purposes only)		
SPECIMIN HANDLING	99000			VARICELLA	90716		PERIODIC ORAL EVALUATION	DE0100	
OFFICE PROCEDURES				LABORATORY			COMPREHENSIVE EVALUATION	DE0150	
ANOSCOPY	46600			VENIPUNCTURE	36415		INTRAORAL, PERIAPICAL – 1ST FILM	DE0200	
AUDIOMETRY	92551			BLOOD GLUCOSE, MONITORING DEVICE	82962		INTRAORAL, PERIAPICAL–EACH ADD'L FILM	DE0250	
CERUMEN REMOVAL	69210			BLOOD GLUCOSE, VISUAL DIPSTICK	82948		BITEWING	DE026-	
COLPOSCOPY	54752			CBC, W/ AUTO DIFFERENTIAL	85025		PROPHYLAXIS - ADULT	DE1000	
COLPOSCOPY W/ BIOPSY	57455			CBC, W/O AUTO DIFFRENTIAL	85027		PROPHYLAXIS - CHILD	DE2000	
ECG W/ INTERPRETATION	93000			CHOLESTEROL	82465		PERIODONTAL MAINT.	DE5000	
ECG, RHYTHM STRIP	93040			HEMOOCULT, GUAIAC	82272		RESTORATIVE (ANTERIOR)	DE250-	
ENDOMETRIAL BIOPSY	58100			HEMOCCULT, IMMUNOASSAY	82274		RESTORATIVE (POSTERIOR)	DE260-	
FLEXIBLE SIGMOIDOSCOPY	45330			HEMOGLOBIN A1C	83036		FUSE CROWN-PORC	DE2700	
FLEXIBLE SIGMOIDOSCOPY W/ BIOPSY	45331			LIPID PANEL	80061		RE-CEMENT CROWN	DE2900	
FRACTURE CARE, CAST/SPLINT	29---			LIVER PANEL	80076		CORE BUILD UP INC. PINS	DE3000	
NEBULIZER	94640			KHO PREP (SKIN, HAIR, NAILS)	87220		CORE BUILD UP, PREFAB POST	DE3250	
NEBULIZER DEMO	94664			METABOLIC PANEL, BASIC	80048		LABIAL VENEER	DE3500	
SPIROMETRY	94010			METABOLIC PANEL, COMPHREHENSIVE	80053		CROWN - PORCELAIN FUSED TO GOLD	DE6000	
SPIROMETRY, PRE AND POST	94060			MONONUCLEOSIS	86663		CROWN LENGTHENING	DE4000	
TYMPANOMETRY	92567			PREGNANCY, BLOOD	84702		SURGICAL EXTRACTION	DE7000	
VASECTOMY	55250			PREGNANCY, URINE	81025		IMPACTED EXTRACTION	DE7250	
MEDICATIONS				RENAL PANEL	80069		LTD. ORTHO TREATMENT, ADULT	DE8000	
AMPICILIN, UP TO 500MG	J0290			SEDIMENTATION RATE	85652		ANALGESIA, NITROUS OXIDE	DE9000	

TODAY'S FEE		70.00
AMOUNT RECEIVED		25.00
BALANCE		45.00

WALDEN-MARTIN
FAMILY MEDICAL CLINIC
1234 ANYSTREET | ANYTOWN, ANYSTATE 12345
PHONE 123-123-1234 | FAX 123-123-5678

JULIE WALDEN MD
JAMES MARTIN MD
DAVID KAHN MD
ANGELA PEREZ MD
PATRICK TAYLOR DDS
JEAN BURKE NP

Patient Name: Reeves, Kyle
DOS: 11/16/15
Diagnoses 1): R10.10
2): R11.0
3):
4):

SERVICE	CODE New	Est.	PRICE	SERVICE	CODE	PRICE	SERVICE	CODE	PRICE
OFFICE VISIT				**MEDICATIONS CONT'D**			**LABORATORY CONT'D**		
MINIMAL OFFICE VISIT (OV)	99201	99211		B-12, UP TO 1,000MCG	J3420		STREP, RAPID	87880	
PROBLEM FOCUSED OV	99202	99212		EPINEPHINE, UP TO 1ML	J0170		STREP CULTURE	87081	
EXPANDED OV	99203	99213		KENALOG, 10MG	J3301		TB	87116	
DETAILED OV	99204	99214		LIDCAINE, 10MG	J2001		UA, COMPLETE, NON-AUTOMATED, MICRO	81000	
COMPREHENSIVE OV	99205	99215		PROGESTERONE, 150MG	J1055		UA, W/O MICRO NON-AUTOMATED	81002	
WELLNESS VISIT	New	Est.		RECEPHIN, 250MG	J0696		UA, W/ MICRO, NON-AUTOMATED	81001	
WELL VISIT < 1 Y	99381	99391		TESTOSTERONE, 200MG	J1080		URINE COLONY COUNT	87086	
WELL VISIT 1-4 Y	99382	99392		TIGAN, UP TO 200MG	J3250		WET MOUNT/KOH	87210	
WELL VISIT 5-11 Y	99383	99393		TORADOL, 15MG	J1885		**INPATIENT/OUTPATIENT PROCEDURES**		
WELL VISIT 12-17 Y	99384	99394		NORMAL SALINE, 1000CC	J7030		UPPER GI ENDOSCOPY	43235	
WELL VISIT 18-39 Y	99385	99395		PHENERGAN, UP TO 50MG	J2550		UPPER GI ENDOSCOPY W/ BIOPSY*	43239	154.00
WELL VISIT 40-64 Y	99386	99396		**IMMUNIZATIONS & INJECTIONS**			UPPER GI ENDOSCOPY W/ GUIDE WIRE	43248	
WELL VISIT 65 Y+	99387	99397		ALLERGEN, ONE	95115		UPPER GI ENDOSCOPY W/ BALLOON	43249	
PREVENTATIVE SERVICES				ALLERGEN, MULTIPLE	95117		COLONOSCOPY	45378	
PAP	Q0091			IMM ADMIN, ONE	90471		COLONOSCOPY W/ BIOPSY	45380	
PELVIC & BREAST	G0101			IMM ADMIN, EACH ADD'L	90472		COLONOSCOPY W/ BIOPSY REMOVAL	45384	
PROSTATE/PSA	G0103			IMM ADMIN, INTRANASAL, ONE	90473		COLONOSCOPY W/ SNARE REMOVAL	45385	
TOBACCO COUNSELING/3-10MIN	99406			IMM ADMIN, INTRANASAL, EACH ADD'L	90475		**SKIN PROCEDURES**		
TOBACCO COUNSELING/>10MIN	99407			INJECTION, JOINT, SMALL	206--		BURN CARE, INITIAL	16000	
WELCOME TO MEDICARE EXAM	G0366			INJECTION, THER/PROPH/DIAG	90772		FROEIGN BODY, SKIN, SIMPLE	10120	
ECG W/ WELCOME TO MEDICARE EXAM	G0366			INJECTION, TRIGGER POINT	20552		FOREIGN BODY, SKIN, COMPLEX	12121	
FLEXIBLE SIGMOIDOSCOPY	G0104			**VACCINES**			I&D, ABSCESS	10060	
HEMOCCULT, GUAIAC	G0107			DT, <7 Y	90702		I&D, HEMATOMA/SEROMA	10140	
FLU ADMINISTRATION	G0008			DTP	90701		LCERATION REPAIR, SIMPLE	120--	
PENUMONIA ADMINISTRATION	G0009			DTAP, <7 Y	90700		LACERATION REPAIR, LAYERED	120--	
CONSULTATION/PRE-OP CLEARANCE				FLU, 6-35 MONTHS	90657		LESION, BIOPSY, ONE	11100	
EXPANDED PROBLEM FOCUSED	99242			FLU, 3Y+	90658		LESION, BIOPSY, EACH ADD'L	11101	
DETAILED	99243			HEP A, PED/ADOL, 2 DOSE	90633		LESION, DEST., BENIGN 1-14	17110	
COMPREHENSIVE/MOD COMPLEXITY	99244			HEP A, ADULT	90632		LESION DEST., PRE-MAL., SINGLE	17000	
COMPREHENSIVE/HIGH COMPLEXITY	99245			HEP B, PED/ADOL, 3 DOSE	90744		LESION DEST., PRE-MAL., EACH ADD'L	17003	
OTHER SERVICES				HEP B, ADULT	90746		LESION, EXCISION BENIGN	114--	
AFTER POSTED HOURS	99050			HEP B-HIB	90748		LESION, EXCISION, MALIGNANT	116--	
EVENING/WEEKEND APPT.	99051			HIB, 4 DOSE	90645		LESION, PARING/CUTTING, ONE	11055	
HOME HEALTH CERTIFICATION	G0180			HPV	90649		LESION PARING/CUTTING 2-4	11056	
HOME HEALTH RECERTIFICATION	G0179			IPV	90713		LESION, SHAVE	113--	
POST-OP FOLLOW UP	99024			MMR	90707		NAIL REMOVAL, PARTIAL	11730	
PROLONGED/30-74MIN	99354			PNEUMONIA, >2 Y	90732		NAIL REMOVAL, W/ MATRIX	11750	
SPECIAL REPORTS/FORMS	99080			PNEUMONIA CONJUGATE, <5Y	90669		SKIN TA, 1-15	11200	
DISABILITY/WORKERS COMP	99455			TD, > 7Y	90718		**DENTAL (For practice purposes only)**		
SPECIMIN HANDLING	99000			VARICELLA	90716		PERIODIC ORAL EVALUATION	DE0100	
OFFICE PROCEDURES				**LABORATORY**			COMPREHENSIVE EVALUATION	DE0150	
ANOSCOPY	46600			VENIPUNCTURE	36415		INTRAORAL, PERIAPICAL – 1ST FILM	DE0200	
AUDIOMETRY	92551			BLOOD GLUCOSE, MONITORING DEVICE	82962		INTRAORAL, PERIAPICAL–EACH ADD'L FILM	DE0250	
CERUMEN REMOVAL	69210			BLOOD GLUCOSE, VISUAL DIPSTICK	82948		BITEWING	DE026-	
COLPOSCOPY	54752			CBC, W/ AUTO DIFFERENTIAL	85025		PROPHYLAXIS - ADULT	DE1000	
COLPOSCOPY W/ BIOPSY	57455			CBC, W/O AUTO DIFFRENTIAL	85027		PROPHYLAXIS - CHILD	DE2000	
ECG W/ INTERPRETATION	93000			CHOLESTEROL	82465		PERIODONTAL MAINT.	DE5000	
ECG, RHYTHM STRIP	93040			HEMOOCULT, GUAIAC	82272		RESTORATIVE (ANTERIOR)	DE250-	
ENDOMETRIAL BIOPSY	58100			HEMOCCULT, IMMUNOASSAY	82274		RESTORATIVE (POSTERIOR)	DE260-	
FLEXIBLE SIGMOIDOSCOPY	45330			HEMOGLOBIN A1C	83036		FUSE CROWN-PORC	DE2700	
FLEXIBLE SIGMOIDOSCOPY W/ BIOPSY	45331			LIPID PANEL	80061		RE-CEMENT CROWN	DE2900	
FRACTURE CARE, CAST/SPLINT	29---			LIVER PANEL	80076		CORE BUILD UP INC. PINS	DE3000	
NEBULIZER	94640			KHO PREP (SKIN, HAIR, NAILS)	87220		CORE BUILD UP, PREFAB POST	DE3250	
NEBULIZER DEMO	94664			METABOLIC PANEL, BASIC	80048		LABIAL VENEER	DE3500	
SPIROMETRY	94010			METABOLIC PANEL, COMPHREHENSIVE	80053		CROWN - PORCELAIN FUSED TO GOLD	DE6000	
SPIROMETRY, PRE AND POST	94060			MONONUCLEOSIS	86663		CROWN LENGTHENING	DE4000	
TYMPANOMETRY	92567			PREGNANCY, BLOOD	84702		SURGICAL EXTRACTION	DE7000	
VASECTOMY	55250			PREGNANCY, URINE	81025		IMPACTED EXTRACTION	DE7250	
MEDICATIONS				RENAL PANEL	80069		LTD. ORTHO TREATMENT, ADULT	DE8000	
AMPICILIN, UP TO 500MG	J0290			SEDIMENTATION RATE	85652		ANALGESIA, NITROUS OXIDE	DE9000	

*Performed at Anytown Outpatient Surgery Center

TODAY'S FEE	154.00
AMOUNT RECEIVED	0.00
BALANCE	154.00

Claim Entry

WALDEN-MARTIN
FAMILY MEDICAL CLINIC
1234 ANYSTREET | ANYTOWN, ANYSTATE 12345
PHONE 123-123-1234 | FAX 123-123-5678

JULIE WALDEN MD
JAMES MARTIN MD
DAVID KAHN MD
ANGELA PEREZ MD
PATRICK TAYLOR DDS
JEAN BURKE NP

Patient Name: Berkley, Julia
DOS: 11/20/2015
Diagnoses 1): Z01.419
2):
3):
4):

SERVICE	CODE New	CODE Est.	PRICE	SERVICE	CODE	PRICE	SERVICE	CODE	PRICE
OFFICE VISIT	New	Est.		**MEDICATIONS CONT'D**			**LABORATORY CONT'D**		
MINIMAL OFFICE VISIT (OV)	99201	99211		B-12, UP TO 1,000MCG	J3420		STREP, RAPID	87880	
PROBLEM FOCUSED OV	99202	99212		EPINEPHINE, UP TO 1ML	J0170		STREP CULTURE	87081	
EXPANDED OV	99203	99213		KENALOG, 10MG	J3301		TB	87116	
DETAILED OV	99204	99214		LIDCAINE, 10MG	J2001		UA, COMPLETE, NON-AUTOMATED, MICRO	81000	
COMPHREHENSIVE OV	99205	99215		PROGESTERONE, 150MG	J1055		UA, W/O MICRO NON-AUTOMATED	81002	
WELLNESS VISIT	New	Est.		RECEPHIN, 250MG	J0696		UA, W/ MICRO, NON-AUTOMATED	81001	
WELL VISIT < 1 Y	99381	99391		TESTOSTERONE, 200MG	J1080		URINE COLONY COUNT	87086	
WELL VISIT 1-4 Y	99382	99392		TIGAN, UP TO 200MG	J3250		WET MOUNT/KOH	87210	
WELL VISIT 5-11 Y	99383	99393		TORADOL, 15MG	J1885		**INPATIENT/OUTPATIENT PROCEDURES**		
WELL VISIT 12-17 Y	99384	99394		NORMAL SALINE, 1000CC	J7030		UPPER GI ENDOSCOPY	43235	
WELL VISIT 18-39 Y	99385	99395		PHENERGAN, UP TO 50MG	J2550		UPPER GI ENDOSCOPY W/ BIOPSY	43239	
WELL VISIT 40-64 Y	99386	99396		**IMMUNIZATIONS & INJECTIONS**			UPPER GI ENDOSCOPY W/ GUIDE WIRE	43248	
WELL VISIT 65 Y+	99387	99397		ALLERGEN, ONE	95115		UPPER GI ENDOSCOPY W/ BALLOON	43249	
PREVENTATIVE SERVICES				ALLERGEN, MULTIPLE	95117		COLONOSCOPY	45378	
PAP	Q0091		79.00	IMM ADMIN, ONE	90471		COLONOSCOPY W/ BIOPSY	45380	
PELVIC & BREAST	G0101		52.00	IMM ADMIN, EACH ADD'L	90472		COLONOSCOPY W/ BIOPSY REMOVAL	45384	
PROSTATE/PSA	G0103			IMM ADMIN, INTRANASAL, ONE	90473		COLONOSCOPY W/ SNARE REMOVAL	45385	
TOBACCO COUNSELING/3-10MIN	99406			IMM ADMIN, INTRANASAL, EACH ADD'L	90475		**SKIN PROCEDURES**		
TOBACCO COUNSELING/>10MIN	99407			INJECTION, JOINT, SMALL	206--		BURN CARE, INITIAL	16000	
WELCOME TO MEDICARE EXAM	G0366			INJECTION, THER/PROPH/DIAG	90772		FROEIGN BODY, SKIN, SIMPLE	10120	
ECG W/ WELCOME TO MEDICARE EXAM	G0366			INJECTION, TRIGGER POINT	20552		FOREIGN BODY, SKIN, COMPLEX	12121	
FLEXIBLE SIGMOIDOSCOPY	G0104			**VACCINES**			I&D, ABSCESS	10060	
HEMOCCULT, GUAIAC	G0107			DT, <7Y	90702		I&D, HEMATOMA/SEROMA	10140	
FLU ADMINISTRATION	G0008			DTP	90701		LCERATION REPAIR, SIMPLE	120--	
PENUMONIA ADMINISTRATION	G0009			DTAP, <7 Y	90700		LACERATION REPAIR, LAYERED	120--	
CONSULTATION/PRE-OP CLEARANCE				FLU, 6-35 MONTHS	90657		LESION, BIOPSY, ONE	11100	
EXPANDED PROBLEM FOCUSED	99242			FLU, 3Y+	90658		LESION, BIOPSY, EACH ADD'L	11101	
DETAILED	99243			HEP A, PED/ADOL, 2 DOSE	90633		LESION, DEST., BENIGN 1-14	17110	
COMPREHENSIVE/MOD COMPLEXITY	99244			HEP A, ADULT	90632		LESION DEST., PRE-MAL., SINGLE	17000	
COMPREHENSIVE/HIGH COMPLEXITY	99245			HEP B, PED/ADOL, 3 DOSE	90744		LESION DEST., PRE-MAL., EACH ADD'L	17003	
OTHER SERVICES				HEP B, ADULT	90746		LESION, EXCISION BENIGN	114--	
AFTER POSTED HOURS	99050			HEP B-HIB	90748		LESION, EXCISION MALIGNANT	116--	
EVENING/WEEKEND APPT.	99051			HIB, 4 DOSE	90645		LESION, PARING/CUTTING, ONE	11055	
HOME HEALTH CERTIFICATION	G0180			HPV	90649		LESION PARING/CUTTING 2-4	11056	
HOME HEALTH RECERTIFICATION	G0179			IPV	90713		LESION, SHAVE	113--	
POST-OP FOLLOW UP	99024			MMR	90707		NAIL REMOVAL, PARTIAL	11730	
PROLONGED/30-74MIN	99354			PNEUMONIA, >2 Y	90732		NAIL REMOVAL, W/ MATRIX	11750	
SPECIAL REPORTS/FORMS	99080			PNEUMONIA CONJUGATE, <5Y	90669		SKIN TA, 1-15	11200	
DISABILITY/WORKERS COMP	99455			TD, > 7Y	90718		**DENTAL (For practice purposes only)**		
SPECIMIN HANDLING	99000			VARICELLA	90716		PERIODIC ORAL EVALUATION	DE0100	
OFFICE PROCEDURES				**LABORATORY**			COMPREHENSIVE EVALUATION	DE0150	
ANOSCOPY	46600			VENIPUNCTURE	36415		INTRAORAL, PERIAPICAL – 1ST FILM	DE0200	
AUDIOMETRY	92551			BLOOD GLUCOSE, MONITORING DEVICE	82962		INTRAORAL, PERIAPICAL–EACH ADD'L FILM	DE0250	
CERUMEN REMOVAL	69210			BLOOD GLUCOSE, VISUAL DIPSTICK	82948		BITEWING	DE026-	
COLPOSCOPY	54752			CBC, W/ AUTO DIFFERENTIAL	85025		PROPHYLAXIS - ADULT	DE1000	
COLPOSCOPY W/ BIOPSY	57455			CBC, W/O AUTO DIFFRENTIAL	85027		PROPHYLAXIS - CHILD	DE2000	
ECG W/ INTERPRETATION	93000			CHOLESTEROL	82465		PERIODONTAL MAINT.	DE5000	
ECG, RHYTHM STRIP	93040			HEMOOCULT, GUAIAC	82272		RESTORATIVE (ANTERIOR)	DE250-	
ENDOMETRIAL BIOPSY	58100			HEMOCULT, IMMUNOASSAY	82274		RESTORATIVE (POSTERIOR)	DE260-	
FLEXIBLE SIGMOIDOSCOPY	45330			HEMOGLOBIN A1C	83036		FUSE CROWN-PORC	DE2700	
FLEXIBLE SIGMOIDOSCOPY W/ BIOPSY	45331			LIPID PANEL	80061		RE-CEMENT CROWN	DE2900	
FRACTURE CARE, CAST/SPLINT	29---			LIVER PANEL	80076		CORE BUILD UP INC. PINS	DE3000	
NEBULIZER	94640			KHO PREP (SKIN, HAIR, NAILS)	87220		CORE BUILD UP, PREFAB POST	DE3250	
NEBULIZER DEMO	94664			METABOLIC PANEL, BASIC	80048		LABIAL VENEER	DE3500	
SPIROMETRY	94010			METABOLIC PANEL, COMPHREHENSIVE	80053		CROWN - PORCELAIN FUSED TO GOLD	DE6000	
SPIROMETRY, PRE AND POST	94060			MONONUCLEOSIS	86663		CROWN LENGTHENING	DE4000	
TYMPANOMETRY	92567			PREGNANCY, BLOOD	84702		SURGICAL EXTRACTION	DE7000	
VASECTOMY	55250			PREGNANCY, URINE	81025		IMPACTED EXTRACTION	DE7250	
MEDICATIONS				RENAL PANEL	80069		LTD. ORTHO TREATMENT, ADULT	DE8000	
AMPICILIN, UP TO 500MG	J0290			SEDIMENTATION RATE	85652		ANALGESIA, NITROUS OXIDE	DE9000	

TODAY'S FEE	131.00
AMOUNT RECEIVED	25.00
BALANCE	106.00

WALDEN-MARTIN
FAMILY MEDICAL CLINIC
1234 ANYSTREET | ANYTOWN, ANYSTATE 12345
PHONE 123-123-1234 | FAX 123-123-5678

JULIE WALDEN MD
JAMES MARTIN MD
DAVID KAHN MD
ANGELA PEREZ MD
PATRICK TAYLOR DDS
JEAN BURKE NP

Patient Name: Ahmad, Reuven
DOS: 11/18/2015
Diagnoses 1): Z00.00
2):
3):
4):

SERVICE	CODE New	Est.	PRICE	SERVICE	CODE	PRICE	SERVICE	CODE	PRICE
OFFICE VISIT	New	Est.		MEDICATIONS CONT'D			LABORATORY CONT'D		
MINIMAL OFFICE VISIT (OV)	99201	99211		B-12, UP TO 1,000MCG	J3420		STREP, RAPID	87880	
PROBLEM FOCUSED OV	99202	99212		EPINEPHINE, UP TO 1ML	J0170		STREP CULTURE	87081	
EXPANDED OV	99203	99213		KENALOG, 10MG	J3301		TB	87116	
DETAILED OV	99204	99214		LIDCAINE, 10MG	J2001		UA, COMPLETE, NON-AUTOMATED, MICRO	81000	
COMPHREHENSIVE OV	99205	99215		PROGESTERONE, 150MG	J1055		UA, W/O MICRO NON-AUTOMATED	81002	
WELLNESS VISIT	New	Est.		RECEPHIN, 250MG	J0696		UA, W/ MICRO, NON-AUTOMATED	81001	27.00
WELL VISIT < 1 Y	99381	99391		TESTOSTERONE, 200MG	J1080		URINE COLONY COUNT	87086	
WELL VISIT 1-4 Y	99382	99392		TIGAN, UP TO 200MG	J3250		WET MOUNT/KOH	87210	
WELL VISIT 5-11 Y	99383	99393		TORADOL, 15MG	J1885		INPATIENT/OUTPATIENT PROCEDURES		
WELL VISIT 12-17 Y	99384	99394		NORMAL SALINE, 1000CC	J7030		UPPER GI ENDOSCOPY	43235	
WELL VISIT 18-39 Y	99385	99395		PHENERGAN, UP TO 50MG	J2550		UPPER GI ENDOSCOPY W/ BIOPSY	43239	
WELL VISIT 40-64 Y	99386	99396	110.00	IMMUNIZATIONS & INJECTIONS			UPPER GI ENDOSCOPY W/ GUIDE WIRE	43248	
WELL VISIT 65 Y+	99387	99397		ALLERGEN, ONE	95115		UPPER GI ENDOSCOPY W/ BALLOON	43249	
PREVENTATIVE SERVICES				ALLERGEN, MULTIPLE	95117		COLONOSCOPY	45378	
PAP	Q0091			IMM ADMIN, ONE	90471		COLONOSCOPY W/ BIOPSY	45380	
PELVIC & BREAST	G0101			IMM ADMIN, EACH ADD'L	90472		COLONOSCOPY W/ BIOPSY REMOVAL	45384	
PROSTATE/PSA	G0103			IMM ADMIN, INTRANASAL, ONE	90473		COLONOSCOPY W/ SNARE REMOVAL	45385	
TOBACCO COUNSELING/3-10MIN	99406			IMM ADMIN, INTRANASAL, EACH ADD'L	90475		SKIN PROCEDURES		
TOBACCO COUNSELING/>10MIN	99407			INJECTION, JOINT, SMALL	206--		BURN CARE, INITIAL	16000	
WELCOME TO MEDICARE EXAM	G0366			INJECTION, THER/PROPH/DIAG	90772		FROEIGN BODY, SKIN, SIMPLE	10120	
ECG W/ WELCOME TO MEDICARE EXAM	G0366			INJECTION, TRIGGER POINT	20552		FOREIGN BODY, SKIN, COMPLEX	12121	
FLEXIBLE SIGMOIDOSCOPY	G0104			VACCINES			I&D, ABSCESS	10060	
HEMOCCULT, GUAIAC	G0107			DT, <7 Y	90702		I&D, HEMATOMA/SEROMA	10140	
FLU ADMINISTRATION	G0008			DTP	90701		LCERATION REPAIR, SIMPLE	120--	
PENUMONIA ADMINISTRATION	G0009			DTAP, <7 Y	90700		LACERATION REPAIR, LAYERED	120--	
CONSULTATION/PRE-OP CLEARANCE				FLU, 6-35 MONTHS	90657		LESION, BIOPSY, ONE	11100	
EXPANDED PROBLEM FOCUSED	99242			FLU, 3Y+	90658		LESION, BIOPSY, EACH ADD'L	11101	
DETAILED	99243			HEP A, PED/ADOL, 2 DOSE	90633		LESION, DEST., BENIGN 1-14	17110	
COMPREHENSIVE/MOD COMPLEXITY	99244			HEP A, ADULT	90632		LESION DEST., PRE-MAL., SINGLE	17000	
COMPREHENSIVE/HIGH COMPLEXITY	99245			HEP B, PED/ADOL, 3 DOSE	90744		LESION DEST., PRE-MAL., EACH ADD'L	17003	
OTHER SERVICES				HEP B, ADULT	90746		LESION, EXCISION BENIGN	114--	
AFTER POSTED HOURS	99050			HEP B-HIB	90748		LESION, EXCISION, MALIGNANT	116--	
EVENING/WEEKEND APPT.	99051			HIB, 4 DOSE	90645		LESION, PARING/CUTTING, ONE	11055	
HOME HEALTH CERTIFICATION	G0180			HPV	90649		LESION PARING/CUTTING 2-4	11056	
HOME HEALTH RECERTIFICATION	G0179			IPV	90713		LESION, SHAVE	113--	
POST-OP FOLLOW UP	99024			MMR	90707		NAIL REMOVAL, PARTIAL	11730	
PROLONGED/30-74MIN	99354			PNEUMONIA, >2 Y	90732		NAIL REMOVAL, W/ MATRIX	11750	
SPECIAL REPORTS/FORMS	99080			PNEUMONIA CONJUGATE, <5Y	90669		SKIN TA, 1-15	11200	
DISABILITY/WORKERS COMP	99455			TD, > 7Y	90718		DENTAL (For practice purposes only)		
SPECIMIN HANDLING	99000			VARICELLA	90716		PERIODIC ORAL EVALUATION	DE0100	
OFFICE PROCEDURES				LABORATORY			COMPREHENSIVE EVALUATION	DE0150	
ANOSCOPY	46600			VENIPUNCTURE	36415		INTRAORAL, PERIAPICAL -- 1ST FILM	DE0200	
AUDIOMETRY	92551			BLOOD GLUCOSE, MONITORING DEVICE	82962		INTRAORAL, PERIAPICAL--EACH ADD'L FILM	DE0250	
CERUMEN REMOVAL	69210			BLOOD GLUCOSE, VISUAL DIPSTICK	82948		BITEWING	DE026-	
COLPOSCOPY	54752			CBC, W/ AUTO DIFFERENTIAL	85025	35.00	PROPHYLAXIS - ADULT	DE1000	
COLPOSCOPY W/ BIOPSY	57455			CBC, W/O AUTO DIFFRENTIAL	85027		PROPHYLAXIS - CHILD	DE2000	
ECG W/ INTERPRETATION	93000	89.00		CHOLESTEROL	82465		PERIODONTAL MAINT.	DE5000	
ECG, RHYTHM STRIP	93040			HEMOOCULT, GUAIAC	82272		RESTORATIVE (ANTERIOR)	DE250-	
ENDOMETRIAL BIOPSY	58100			HEMOCCULT, IMMUNOASSAY	82274		RESTORATIVE (POSTERIOR)	DE260-	
FLEXIBLE SIGMOIDOSCOPY	45330			HEMOGLOBIN A1C	83036		FUSE CROWN-PORC	DE2700	
FLEXIBLE SIGMOIDOSCOPY W/ BIOPSY	45331			LIPID PANEL	80061		RE-CEMENT CROWN	DE2900	
FRACTURE CARE, CAST/SPLINT	29---			LIVER PANEL	80076		CORE BUILD UP INC. PINS	DE3000	
NEBULIZER	94640			KHO PREP (SKIN, HAIR, NAILS)	87220		CORE BUILD UP, PREFAB POST	DE3250	
NEBULIZER DEMO	94664			METABOLIC PANEL, BASIC	80048		LABIAL VENEER	DE3500	
SPIROMETRY	94010			METABOLIC PANEL, COMPHREHENSIVE	80053		CROWN - PORCELAIN FUSED TO GOLD	DE6000	
SPIROMETRY, PRE AND POST	94060			MONONUCLEOSIS	86663		CROWN LENGTHENING	DE4000	
TYMPANOMETRY	92567			PREGNANCY, BLOOD	84702		SURGICAL EXTRACTION	DE7000	
VASECTOMY	55250			PREGNANCY, URINE	81025		IMPACTED EXTRACTION	DE7250	
MEDICATIONS				RENAL PANEL	80069		LTD. ORTHO TREATMENT, ADULT	DE8000	
AMPICILIN, UP TO 500MG	J0290			SEDIMENTATION RATE	85652		ANALGESIA, NITROUS OXIDE	DE9000	

TODAY'S FEE		261.00
AMOUNT RECEIVED		25.00
BALANCE		236.00

Claim Entry

WALDEN-MARTIN
FAMILY MEDICAL CLINIC
1234 ANYSTREET | ANYTOWN, ANYSTATE 12345
PHONE 123-123-1234 | FAX 123-123-5678

JULIE WALDEN MD
JAMES MARTIN MD
DAVID KAHN MD
ANGELA PEREZ MD
PATRICK TAYLOR DDS
JEAN BURKE NP

Patient Name: Rodriguez, Noemi
DOS: 11/16/2015
Diagnoses 1):
2):
3):
4):

SERVICE	CODE		PRICE	SERVICE	CODE	PRICE	SERVICE	CODE	PRICE
OFFICE VISIT	**New**	**Est.**		**MEDICATIONS CONT'D**			**LABORATORY CONT'D**		
MINIMAL OFFICE VISIT (OV)	99201	99211		B-12, UP TO 1,000MCG	J3420		STREP, RAPID	87880	
PROBLEM FOCUSED OV	99202	99212		EPINEPHINE, UP TO 1ML	J0170		STREP CULTURE	87081	
EXPANDED OV	99203	99213		KENALOG, 10MG	J3301		TB	87116	
DETAILED OV	99204	99214		LIDCAINE, 10MG	J2001		UA, COMPLETE, NON-AUTOMATED, MICRO	81000	
COMPHREHENSIVE OV	99205	99215		PROGESTERONE, 150MG	J1055		UA, W/O MICRO NON-AUTOMATED	81002	
WELLNESS VISIT	**New**	**Est.**		RECEPHIN, 250MG	J0696		UA, W/ MICRO, NON-AUTOMATED	81001	
WELL VISIT < 1 Y	99381	99391		TESTOSTERONE, 200MG	J1080		URINE COLONY COUNT	87086	
WELL VISIT 1-4 Y	99382	99392		TIGAN, UP TO 200MG	J3250		WET MOUNT/KOH	87210	
WELL VISIT 5-11 Y	99383	99393		TORADOL, 15MG	J1885		**INPATIENT/OUTPATIENT PROCEDURES**		
WELL VISIT 12-17 Y	99384	99394		NORMAL SALINE, 1000CC	J7030		UPPER GI ENDOSCOPY	43235	
WELL VISIT 18-39 Y	99385	99395		PHENERGAN, UP TO 50MG	J2550		UPPER GI ENDOSCOPY W/ BIOPSY	43239	
WELL VISIT 40-64 Y	99386	99396		**IMMUNIZATIONS & INJECTIONS**			UPPER GI ENDOSCOPY W/ GUIDE WIRE	43248	
WELL VISIT 65 Y+	99387	99397		ALLERGEN, ONE	95115		UPPER GI ENDOSCOPY W/ BALLOON	43249	
PREVENTATIVE SERVICES				ALLERGEN, MULTIPLE	95117		COLONOSCOPY	45378	
PAP	Q0091			IMM ADMIN, ONE	90471		COLONOSCOPY W/ BIOPSY	45380	
PELVIC & BREAST	G0101			IMM ADMIN, EACH ADD'L	90472		COLONOSCOPY W/ BIOPSY REMOVAL	45384	
PROSTATE/PSA	G0103			IMM ADMIN, INTRANASAL, ONE	90473		COLONOSCOPY W/ SNARE REMOVAL	45385	
TOBACCO COUNSELING/3-10MIN	99406			IMM ADMIN, INTRANASAL, EACH ADD'L	90475		**SKIN PROCEDURES**		
TOBACCO COUNSELING/>10MIN	99407			INJECTION, JOINT, SMALL	206--		BURN CARE, INITIAL	16000	
WELCOME TO MEDICARE EXAM	G0366			INJECTION, THER/PROPH/DIAG	90772		FROEIGN BODY, SKIN, SIMPLE	10120	
ECG W/ WELCOME TO MEDICARE EXAM	G0366			INJECTION, TRIGGER POINT	20552		FOREIGN BODY, SKIN, COMPLEX	12121	
FLEXIBLE SIGMOIDOSCOPY	G0104			**VACCINES**			I&D, ABSCESS	10060	
HEMOCCULT, GUAIAC	G0107			DT, <7 Y	90702		I&D, HEMATOMA/SEROMA	10140	
FLU ADMINISTRATION	G0008			DTP	90701		LCERATION REPAIR, SIMPLE	120--	
PENUMONIA ADMINISTRATION	G0009			DTAP, <7 Y	90700		LACERATION REPAIR, LAYERED	120--	
CONSULTATION/PRE-OP CLEARANCE				FLU, 6-35 MONTHS	90657		LESION, BIOPSY, ONE	11100	
EXPANDED PROBLEM FOCUSED	99242			FLU, 3Y+	90658		LESION, BIOPSY, EACH ADD'L	11101	
DETAILED	99243			HEP A, PED/ADOL, 2 DOSE	90633		LESION, DEST., BENIGN 1-14	17110	
COMPREHENSIVE/MOD COMPLEXITY	99244			HEP A, ADULT	90632		LESION DEST., PRE-MAL., SINGLE	17000	
COMPREHENSIVE/HIGH COMPLEXITY	99245			HEP B, PED/ADOL, 3 DOSE	90744		LESION DEST., PRE-MAL., EACH ADD'L	17003	
OTHER SERVICES				HEP B, ADULT	90746		LESION, EXCISION BENIGN	114--	
AFTER POSTED HOURS	99050			HEP B-HIB	90748		LESION, EXCISION, MALIGNANT	116--	
EVENING/WEEKEND APPT.	99051			HIB, 4 DOSE	90645		LESION, PARING/CUTTING, ONE	11055	
HOME HEALTH CERTIFICATION	G0180			HPV	90649		LESION PARING/CUTTING 2-4	11056	
HOME HEALTH RECERTIFICATION	G0179			IPV	90713		LESION, SHAVE	113--	
POST-OP FOLLOW UP	99024			MMR	90707		NAIL REMOVAL, PARTIAL	11730	
PROLONGED/30-74MIN	99354			PNEUMONIA, >2 Y	90732		NAIL REMOVAL, W/ MATRIX	11750	
SPECIAL REPORTS/FORMS	99080			PNEUMONIA CONJUGATE, <5Y	90669		SKIN TA, 1-15	11200	
DISABILITY/WORKERS COMP	99455			TD, > 7Y	90718		**DENTAL (For practice purposes only)**		
SPECIMIN HANDLING	99000			VARICELLA	90716		PERIODIC ORAL EVALUATION	DE0100	
OFFICE PROCEDURES				**LABORATORY**			COMPREHENSIVE EVALUATION	DE0150	
ANOSCOPY	46600			VENIPUNCTURE	36415		INTRAORAL, PERIAPICAL – 1ST FILM	DE0200	
AUDIOMETRY	92551			BLOOD GLUCOSE, MONITORING DEVICE	82962		INTRAORAL, PERIAPICAL--EACH ADD'L FILM	DE0250	
CERUMEN REMOVAL	69210			BLOOD GLUCOSE, VISUAL DIPSTICK	82948		BITEWING	DE026-	
COLPOSCOPY	54752			CBC, W/ AUTO DIFFERENTIAL	85025		PROPHYLAXIS - ADULT	DE1000	64.00
COLPOSCOPY W/ BIOPSY	57455			CBC, W/O AUTO DIFFRENTIAL	85027		PROPHYLAXIS - CHILD	DE2000	
ECG W/ INTERPRETATION	93000			CHOLESTEROL	82465		PERIODONTAL MAINT.	DE5000	
ECG, RHYTHM STRIP	93040			HEMOOCULT, GUAIAC	82272		RESTORATIVE (ANTERIOR)	DE250-	
ENDOMETRIAL BIOPSY	58100			HEMOCCULT, IMMUNOASSAY	82274		RESTORATIVE (POSTERIOR)	DE260-	
FLEXIBLE SIGMOIDOSCOPY	45330			HEMOGLOBIN A1C	83036		FUSE CROWN-PORC	DE2700	
FLEXIBLE SIGMOIDOSCOPY W/ BIOPSY	45331			LIPID PANEL	80061		RE-CEMENT CROWN	DE2900	
FRACTURE CARE, CAST/SPLINT	29---			LIVER PANEL	80076		CORE BUILD UP INC. PINS	DE3000	
NEBULIZER	94640			KHO PREP (SKIN, HAIR, NAILS)	87220		CORE BUILD UP, PREFAB POST	DE3250	
NEBULIZER DEMO	94664			METABOLIC PANEL, BASIC	80048		LABIAL VENEER	DE3500	
SPIROMETRY	94010			METABOLIC PANEL, COMPHREHENSIVE	80053		CROWN - PORCELAIN FUSED TO GOLD	DE6000	
SPIROMETRY, PRE AND POST	94060			MONONUCLEOSIS	86663		CROWN LENGTHENING	DE4000	
TYMPANOMETRY	92567			PREGNANCY, BLOOD	84702		SURGICAL EXTRACTION	DE7000	
VASECTOMY	55250			PREGNANCY, URINE	81025		IMPACTED EXTRACTION	DE7250	
MEDICATIONS				RENAL PANEL	80069		LTD. ORTHO TREATMENT, ADULT	DE8000	
AMPICILIN, UP TO 500MG	J0290			SEDIMENTATION RATE	85652		ANALGESIA, NITROUS OXIDE	DE9000	

TODAY'S FEE		64.00
AMOUNT RECEIVED		0.00
BALANCE		64.00

WALDEN-MARTIN
FAMILY MEDICAL CLINIC
1234 ANYSTREET | ANYTOWN, ANYSTATE 12345
PHONE 123-123-1234 | FAX 123-123-5678

JULIE WALDEN MD
JAMES MARTIN MD
DAVID KAHN MD
ANGELA PEREZ MD
PATRICK TAYLOR DDS
JEAN BURKE NP

PATIENT INFO

First Name	MI	Last Name		Date of Birth	Sex
Noemi		Rodriguez			F

SSN	Preferred Phone	Dental Insurance	Responsible Party
		Self-Pay	Self

BRIEF HISTORY

Last Visit	Treatment	X-Rays: Ⓨ / N
5/5/15	Cleaning	

CLINICAL DATA

General Condition of Teeth
Sensitive to hot/cold

General Condition of Gums
Normal

General Condition of the Floor of the Mouth
Normal

Examination and treatment plan—List in order from tooth no. 1 through no. 32—Use charting system shown

Identify missing teeth with "x"

Tooth # or letter	Surface	Description of service (including x-ray, prophylaxis, materials used, etc.)	Date service performed Mo./Day/Year	Procedure number

Remarks for unusual services

Follow up:
6 Months

Claim Entry

WALDEN-MARTIN
FAMILY MEDICAL CLINIC
1234 ANYSTREET | ANYTOWN, ANYSTATE 12345
PHONE 123-123-1234 | FAX 123-123-5678

JULIE WALDEN MD
JAMES MARTIN MD
DAVID KAHN MD
ANGELA PEREZ MD
PATRICK TAYLOR DDS
JEAN BURKE NP

Patient Name: Burgel, Isabella
DOS: 11/13/2015
Diagnoses 1): K63.5
2):
3):
4):

SERVICE	CODE		PRICE	SERVICE	CODE	PRICE	SERVICE	CODE	PRICE
OFFICE VISIT	New	Est.		**MEDICATIONS CONT'D**			**LABORATORY CONT'D**		
MINIMAL OFFICE VISIT (OV)	99201	99211		B-12, UP TO 1,000MCG	J3420		STREP, RAPID	87880	
PROBLEM FOCUSED OV	99202	99212		EPINEPHINE, UP TO 1ML	J0170		STREP CULTURE	87081	
EXPANDED OV	99203	99213		KENALOG, 10MG	J3301		TB	87116	
DETAILED OV	99204	99214		LIDCAINE, 10MG	J2001		UA, COMPLETE, NON-AUTOMATED, MICRO	81000	
COMPHREHENSIVE OV	99205	99215		PROGESTERONE, 150MG	J1055		UA, W/O MICRO NON-AUTOMATED	81002	
WELLNESS VISIT	New	Est.		RECEPHIN, 250MG	J0696		UA, W/ MICRO, NON-AUTOMATED	81001	
WELL VISIT < 1 Y	99381	99391		TESTOSTERONE, 200MG	J1080		URINE COLONY COUNT	87086	
WELL VISIT 1-4 Y	99382	99392		TIGAN, UP TO 200MG	J3250		WET MOUNT/KOH	87210	
WELL VISIT 5-11 Y	99383	99393		TORADOL, 15MG	J1885		**INPATIENT/OUTPATIENT PROCEDURES**		
WELL VISIT 12-17 Y	99384	99394		NORMAL SALINE, 1000CC	J7030		UPPER GI ENDOSCOPY	43235	
WELL VISIT 18-39 Y	99385	99395		PHENERGAN, UP TO 50MG	J2550		UPPER GI ENDOSCOPY W/ BIOPSY	43239	
WELL VISIT 40-64 Y	99386	99396		**IMMUNIZATIONS & INJECTIONS**			UPPER GI ENDOSCOPY W/ GUIDE WIRE	43248	
WELL VISIT 65 Y+	99387	99397		ALLERGEN, ONE	95115		UPPER GI ENDOSCOPY W/ BALLOON	43249	
PREVENTATIVE SERVICES				ALLERGEN, MULTIPLE	95117		COLONOSCOPY	45378	
PAP	Q0091			IMM ADMIN, ONE	90471		COLONOSCOPY W/ BIOPSY *	45380	265.00
PELVIC & BREAST	G0101			IMM ADMIN, EACH ADD'L	90472		COLONOSCOPY W/ BIOPSY REMOVAL	45384	
PROSTATE/PSA	G0103			IMM ADMIN, INTRANASAL, ONE	90473		COLONOSCOPY W/ SNARE REMOVAL	45385	
TOBACCO COUNSELING/3-10MIN	99406			IMM ADMIN, INTRANASAL, EACH ADD'L	90475		**SKIN PROCEDURES**		
TOBACCO COUNSELING/>10MIN	99407			INJECTION, JOINT, SMALL	206--		BURN CARE, INITIAL	16000	
WELCOME TO MEDICARE EXAM	G0366			INJECTION, THER/PROPH/DIAG	90772		FROEIGN BODY, SKIN, SIMPLE	10120	
ECG W/ WELCOME TO MEDICARE EXAM	G0366			INJECTION, TRIGGER POINT	20552		FOREIGN BODY, SKIN, COMPLEX	12121	
FLEXIBLE SIGMOIDOSCOPY	G0104			**VACCINES**			I&D, ABSCESS	10060	
HEMOCCULT, GUAIAC	G0107			DT, <7 Y	90702		I&D, HEMATOMA/SEROMA	10140	
FLU ADMINISTRATION	G0008			DTP	90701		LCERATION REPAIR, SIMPLE	120--	
PENUMONIA ADMINISTRATION	G0009			DTAP, <7 Y	90700		LACERATION REPAIR, LAYERED	120--	
CONSULTATION/PRE-OP CLEARANCE				FLU, 6-35 MONTHS	90657		LESION, BIOPSY, ONE	11100	
EXPANDED PROBLEM FOCUSED	99242			FLU, 3Y+	90658		LESION, BIOPSY, EACH ADD'L	11101	
DETAILED	99243			HEP A, PED/ADOL, 2 DOSE	90633		LESION, DEST., BENIGN 1-14	17110	
COMPREHENSIVE/MOD COMPLEXITY	99244			HEP A, ADULT	90632		LESION DEST., PRE-MAL., SINGLE	17000	
COMPREHENSIVE/HIGH COMPLEXITY	99245			HEP B, PED/ADOL, 3 DOSE	90744		LESION DEST., PRE-MAL., EACH ADD'L	17003	
OTHER SERVICES				HEP B, ADULT	90746		LESION, EXCISION BENIGN	114--	
AFTER POSTED HOURS	99050			HEP B-HIB	90748		LESION, EXCISION, MALIGNANT	116--	
EVENING/WEEKEND APPT.	99051			HIB, 4 DOSE	90645		LESION, PARING/CUTTING, ONE	11055	
HOME HEALTH CERTIFICATION	G0180			HPV	90649		LESION PARING/CUTTING 2-4	11056	
HOME HEALTH RECERTIFICATION	G0179			IPV	90713		LESION, SHAVE	113--	
POST-OP FOLLOW UP	99024			MMR	90707		NAIL REMOVAL, PARTIAL	11730	
PROLONGED/30-74MIN	99354			PNEUMONIA, >2 Y	90732		NAIL REMOVAL, W/ MATRIX	11750	
SPECIAL REPORTS/FORMS	99080			PNEUMONIA CONJUGATE, <5Y	90669		SKIN TA, 1-15	11200	
DISABILITY/WORKERS COMP	99455			TD, > 7Y	90718		**DENTAL (For practice purposes only)**		
SPECIMIN HANDLING	99000			VARICELLA	90716		PERIODIC ORAL EVALUATION	DE0100	
OFFICE PROCEDURES				**LABORATORY**			COMPREHENSIVE EVALUATION	DE0150	
ANOSCOPY	46600			VENIPUNCTURE	36415		INTRAORAL, PERIAPICAL – 1ST FILM	DE0200	
AUDIOMETRY	92551			BLOOD GLUCOSE, MONITORING DEVICE	82962		INTRAORAL, PERIAPICAL–EACH ADD'L FILM	DE0250	
CERUMEN REMOVAL	69210			BLOOD GLUCOSE, VISUAL DIPSTICK	82948		BITEWING	DE026-	
COLPOSCOPY	54752			CBC, W/ AUTO DIFFERENTIAL	85025		PROPHYLAXIS - ADULT	DE1000	
COLPOSCOPY W/ BIOPSY	57455			CBC, W/O AUTO DIFFRENTIAL	85027		PROPHYLAXIS - CHILD	DE2000	
ECG W/ INTERPRETATION	93000			CHOLESTEROL	82465		PERIODONTAL MAINT.	DE5000	
ECG, RHYTHM STRIP	93040			HEMOOCULT, GUAIAC	82272		RESTORATIVE (ANTERIOR)	DE250-	
ENDOMETRIAL BIOPSY	58100			HEMOCCULT, IMMUNOASSAY	82274		RESTORATIVE (POSTERIOR)	DE260-	
FLEXIBLE SIGMOIDOSCOPY	45330			HEMOGLOBIN A1C	83036		FUSE CROWN-PORC	DE2700	
FLEXIBLE SIGMOIDOSCOPY W/ BIOPSY	45331			LIPID PANEL	80061		RE-CEMENT CROWN	DE2900	
FRACTURE CARE, CAST/SPLINT	29---			LIVER PANEL	80076		CORE BUILD UP INC. PINS	DE3000	
NEBULIZER	94640			KHO PREP (SKIN, HAIR, NAILS)	87220		CORE BUILD UP, PREFAB POST	DE3250	
NEBULIZER DEMO	94664			METABOLIC PANEL, BASIC	80048		LABIAL VENEER	DE3500	
SPIROMETRY	94010			METABOLIC PANEL, COMPHREHENSIVE	80053		CROWN - PORCELAIN FUSED TO GOLD	DE6000	
SPIROMETRY, PRE AND POST	94060			MONONUCLEOSIS	86663		CROWN LENGTHENING	DE4000	
TYMPANOMETRY	92567			PREGNANCY, BLOOD	84702		SURGICAL EXTRACTION	DE7000	
VASECTOMY	55250			PREGNANCY, URINE	81025		IMPACTED EXTRACTION	DE7250	
MEDICATIONS				RENAL PANEL	80069		LTD. ORTHO TREATMENT, ADULT	DE8000	
AMPICILIN, UP TO 500MG	J0290			SEDIMENTATION RATE	85652		ANALGESIA, NITROUS OXIDE	DE9000	

*Performed at Anytown Hospital

TODAY'S FEE	265.00
AMOUNT RECEIVED	0.00
BALANCE	265.00

WALDEN-MARTIN

FAMILY MEDICAL CLINIC
1234 ANYSTREET | ANYTOWN, ANYSTATE 12345
PHONE 123-123-1234 | FAX 123-123-5678

JULIE WALDEN MD
JAMES MARTIN MD
(DAVID KAHN MD)
ANGELA PEREZ MD
PATRICK TAYLOR DDS
JEAN BURKE NP

Patient Name: Gomez, Pedro
DOS: 11/16/2015
Diagnoses 1): B07.9
2):
3):
4):

SERVICE	CODE		PRICE	SERVICE	CODE	PRICE	SERVICE	CODE	PRICE
OFFICE VISIT	New	Est.		MEDICATIONS CONT'D			LABORATORY CONT'D		
MINIMAL OFFICE VISIT (OV)	99201	99211		B-12, UP TO 1,000MCG	J3420		STREP, RAPID	87880	
PROBLEM FOCUSED OV	99202	99212		EPINEPHINE, UP TO 1ML	J0170		STREP CULTURE	87081	
EXPANDED OV	99203	99213		KENALOG, 10MG	J3301		TB	87116	
DETAILED OV	99204	99214		LIDCAINE, 10MG	J2001		UA, COMPLETE, NON-AUTOMATED, MICRO	81000	
COMPHREHENSIVE OV	99205	99215		PROGESTERONE, 150MG	J1055		UA, W/O MICRO NON-AUTOMATED	81002	
WELLNESS VISIT	New	Est.		RECEPHIN, 250MG	J0696		UA, W/ MICRO, NON-AUTOMATED	81001	
WELL VISIT < 1 Y	99381	99391		TESTOSTERONE, 200MG	J1080		URINE COLONY COUNT	87086	
WELL VISIT 1-4 Y	99382	99392		TIGAN, UP TO 200MG	J3250		WET MOUNT/KOH	87210	
WELL VISIT 5-11 Y	99383	99393		TORADOL, 15MG	J1885		INPATIENT/OUTPATIENT PROCEDURES		
WELL VISIT 12-17 Y	99384	99394		NORMAL SALINE, 1000CC	J7030		UPPER GI ENDOSCOPY	43235	
WELL VISIT 18-39 Y	99385	99395		PHENERGAN, UP TO 50MG	J2550		UPPER GI ENDOSCOPY W/ BIOPSY	43239	
WELL VISIT 40-64 Y	99386	99396		IMMUNIZATIONS & INJECTIONS			UPPER GI ENDOSCOPY W/ GUIDE WIRE	43248	
WELL VISIT 65 Y+	99387	99397		ALLERGEN, ONE	95115		UPPER GI ENDOSCOPY W/ BALLOON	43249	
PREVENTATIVE SERVICES				ALLERGEN, MULTIPLE	95117		COLONOSCOPY	45378	
PAP	Q0091			IMM ADMIN, ONE	90471		COLONOSCOPY W/ BIOPSY	45380	
PELVIC & BREAST	G0101			IMM ADMIN, EACH ADD'L	90472		COLONOSCOPY W/ BIOPSY REMOVAL	45384	
PROSTATE/PSA	G0103			IMM ADMIN, INTRANASAL, ONE	90473		COLONOSCOPY W/ SNARE REMOVAL	45385	
TOBACCO COUNSELING/3-10MIN	99406			IMM ADMIN, INTRANASAL, EACH ADD'L	90475		SKIN PROCEDURES		
TOBACCO COUNSELING/>10MIN	99407			INJECTION, JOINT, SMALL	206--		BURN CARE, INITIAL	16000	
WELCOME TO MEDICARE EXAM	G0366			INJECTION, THER/PROPH/DIAG	90772		FROEIGN BODY, SKIN, SIMPLE	10120	
ECG W/ WELCOME TO MEDICARE EXAM	G0366			INJECTION, TRIGGER POINT	20552		FOREIGN BODY, SKIN, COMPLEX	12121	
FLEXIBLE SIGMOIDOSCOPY	G0104			VACCINES			I&D, ABSCESS	10060	
HEMOCCULT, GUAIAC	G0107			DT, <7 Y	90702		I&D, HEMATOMA/SEROMA	10140	
FLU ADMINISTRATION	G0008			DTP	90701		LCERATION REPAIR, SIMPLE	120--	
PENUMONIA ADMINISTRATION	G0009			DTAP, <7 Y	90700		LACERATION REPAIR, LAYERED	120--	
CONSULTATION/PRE-OP CLEARANCE				FLU, 6-35 MONTHS	90657		LESION, BIOPSY, ONE	11100	
EXPANDED PROBLEM FOCUSED	99242			FLU, 3Y+	90658		LESION, BIOPSY, EACH ADD'L	11101	
DETAILED	99243			HEP A, PED/ADOL, 2 DOSE	90633		LESION, DEST., BENIGN 1-14 x8 (17110)		38.00
COMPREHENSIVE/MOD COMPLEXITY	99244			HEP A, ADULT	90632		LESION DEST., PRE-MAL., SINGLE	17000	
COMPREHENSIVE/HIGH COMPLEXITY	99245			HEP B, PED/ADOL, 3 DOSE	90744		LESION DEST., PRE-MAL., EACH ADD'L	17003	
OTHER SERVICES				HEP B, ADULT	90746		LESION, EXCISION BENIGN	114--	
AFTER POSTED HOURS	99050			HEP B-HIB	90748		LESION, EXCISION, MALIGNANT	116--	
EVENING/WEEKEND APPT.	99051			HIB, 4 DOSE	90645		LESION, PARING/CUTTING, ONE	11055	
HOME HEALTH CERTIFICATION	G0180			HPV	90649		LESION PARING/CUTTING 2-4	11056	
HOME HEALTH RECERTIFICATION	G0179			IPV	90713		LESION, SHAVE	113--	
POST-OP FOLLOW UP	99024			MMR	90707		NAIL REMOVAL, PARTIAL	11730	
PROLONGED/30-74MIN	99354			PNEUMONIA, >2 Y	90732		NAIL REMOVAL, W/ MATRIX	11750	
SPECIAL REPORTS/FORMS	99080			PNEUMONIA CONJUGATE, <5Y	90669		SKIN TA, 1-15	11200	
DISABILITY/WORKERS COMP	99455			TD, > 7Y	90718		DENTAL (For practice purposes only)		
SPECIMIN HANDLING	99000			VARICELLA	90716		PERIODIC ORAL EVALUATION	DE0100	
OFFICE PROCEDURES				LABORATORY			COMPREHENSIVE EVALUATION	DE0150	
ANOSCOPY	46600			VENIPUNCTURE	36415		INTRAORAL, PERIAPICAL – 1ST FILM	DE0200	
AUDIOMETRY	92551			BLOOD GLUCOSE, MONITORING DEVICE	82962		INTRAORAL, PERIAPICAL--EACH ADD'L FILM	DE0250	
CERUMEN REMOVAL	69210			BLOOD GLUCOSE, VISUAL DIPSTICK	82948		BITEWING	DE026-	
COLPOSCOPY	54752			CBC, W/ AUTO DIFFERENTIAL	85025		PROPHYLAXIS - ADULT	DE1000	
COLPOSCOPY W/ BIOPSY	57455			CBC, W/O AUTO DIFFRENTIAL	85027		PROPHYLAXIS - CHILD	DE2000	
ECG W/ INTERPRETATION	93000			CHOLESTEROL	82465		PERIODONTAL MAINT.	DE5000	
ECG, RHYTHM STRIP	93040			HEMOOCULT, GUAIAC	82272		RESTORATIVE (ANTERIOR)	DE250-	
ENDOMETRIAL BIOPSY	58100			HEMOCCULT, IMMUNOASSAY	82274		RESTORATIVE (POSTERIOR)	DE260-	
FLEXIBLE SIGMOIDOSCOPY	45330			HEMOGLOBIN A1C	83036		FUSE CROWN-PORC	DE2700	
FLEXIBLE SIGMOIDOSCOPY W/ BIOPSY	45331			LIPID PANEL	80061		RE-CEMENT CROWN	DE2900	
FRACTURE CARE, CAST/SPLINT	29---			LIVER PANEL	80076		CORE BUILD UP INC. PINS	DE3000	
NEBULIZER	94640			KHO PREP (SKIN, HAIR, NAILS)	87220		CORE BUILD UP, PREFAB POST	DE3250	
NEBULIZER DEMO	94664			METABOLIC PANEL, BASIC	80048		LABIAL VENEER	DE3500	
SPIROMETRY	94010			METABOLIC PANEL, COMPHREHENSIVE	80053		CROWN - PORCELAIN FUSED TO GOLD	DE6000	
SPIROMETRY, PRE AND POST	94060			MONONUCLEOSIS	86663		CROWN LENGTHENING	DE4000	
TYMPANOMETRY	92567			PREGNANCY, BLOOD	84702		SURGICAL EXTRACTION	DE7000	
VASECTOMY	55250			PREGNANCY, URINE	81025		IMPACTED EXTRACTION	DE7250	
MEDICATIONS				RENAL PANEL	80069		LTD. ORTHO TREATMENT, ADULT	DE8000	
AMPICILIN, UP TO 500MG	J0290			SEDIMENTATION RATE	85652		ANALGESIA, NITROUS OXIDE	DE9000	

TODAY'S FEE		304.00
AMOUNT RECEIVED		35.00
BALANCE		269.00

Claim Entry

WALDEN-MARTIN
FAMILY MEDICAL CLINIC
1234 ANYSTREET | ANYTOWN, ANYSTATE 12345
PHONE 123-123-1234 | FAX 123-123-5678

JULIE WALDEN MD
JAMES MARTIN MD
DAVID KAHN MD
ANGELA PEREZ MD
PATRICK TAYLOR DDS
JEAN BURKE NP

Patient Name: Green, Jana
DOS: 11/20/15
Diagnoses 1): R11.2
2):
3):
4):

SERVICE	CODE		PRICE	SERVICE	CODE	PRICE	SERVICE	CODE	PRICE
OFFICE VISIT	New	Est.		MEDICATIONS CONT'D			LABORATORY CONT'D		
MINIMAL OFFICE VISIT (OV)	99201	99211		B-12, UP TO 1,000MCG	J3420		STREP, RAPID	87880	
PROBLEM FOCUSED OV	99202	99212		EPINEPHINE, UP TO 1ML	J0170		STREP CULTURE	87081	
EXPANDED OV	99203	99213	70.00	KENALOG, 10MG	J3301		TB	87116	
DETAILED OV	99204	99214		LIDCAINE, 10MG	J2001		UA, COMPLETE, NON-AUTOMATED, MICRO	81000	
COMPHREHENSIVE OV	99205	99215		PROGESTERONE, 150MG	J1055		UA, W/O MICRO NON-AUTOMATED	81002	
WELLNESS VISIT	New	Est.		RECEPHIN, 250MG	J0696		UA, W/ MICRO, NON-AUTOMATED	81001	
WELL VISIT < 1 Y	99381	99391		TESTOSTERONE, 200MG	J1080		URINE COLONY COUNT	87086	
WELL VISIT 1-4 Y	99382	99392		TIGAN, UP TO 200MG	J3250		WET MOUNT/KOH	87210	
WELL VISIT 5-11 Y	99383	99393		TORADOL, 15MG	J1885		INPATIENT/OUTPATIENT PROCEDURES		
WELL VISIT 12-17 Y	99384	99394		NORMAL SALINE, 1000CC	J7030		UPPER GI ENDOSCOPY	43235	
WELL VISIT 18-39 Y	99385	99395		PHENERGAN, UP TO 50MG	J2550		UPPER GI ENDOSCOPY W/ BIOPSY	43239	
WELL VISIT 40-64 Y	99386	99396		IMMUNIZATIONS & INJECTIONS			UPPER GI ENDOSCOPY W/ GUIDE WIRE	43248	
WELL VISIT 65 Y+	99387	99397		ALLERGEN, ONE	95115		UPPER GI ENDOSCOPY W/ BALLOON	43249	
PREVENTATIVE SERVICES				ALLERGEN, MULTIPLE	95117		COLONOSCOPY	45378	
PAP	Q0091			IMM ADMIN, ONE	90471		COLONOSCOPY W/ BIOPSY	45380	
PELVIC & BREAST	G0101			IMM ADMIN, EACH ADD'L	90472		COLONOSCOPY W/ BIOPSY REMOVAL	45384	
PROSTATE/PSA	G0103			IMM ADMIN, INTRANASAL, ONE	90473		COLONOSCOPY W/ SNARE REMOVAL	45385	
TOBACCO COUNSELING/3-10MIN	99406			IMM ADMIN, INTRANASAL, EACH ADD'L	90475		SKIN PROCEDURES		
TOBACCO COUNSELING/>10MIN	99407			INJECTION, JOINT, SMALL	206--		BURN CARE, INITIAL	16000	
WELCOME TO MEDICARE EXAM	G0366			INJECTION, THER/PROPH/DIAG	90772		FROEIGN BODY, SKIN, SIMPLE	10120	
ECG W/ WELCOME TO MEDICARE EXAM	G0366			INJECTION, TRIGGER POINT	20552		FOREIGN BODY, SKIN, COMPLEX	12121	
FLEXIBLE SIGMOIDOSCOPY	G0104			VACCINES			I&D, ABSCESS	10060	
HEMOCCULT, GUAIAC	G0107			DT, <7 Y	90702		I&D, HEMATOMA/SEROMA	10140	
FLU ADMINISTRATION	G0008			DTP	90701		LCERATION REPAIR, SIMPLE	120--	
PENUMONIA ADMINISTRATION	G0009			DTAP, <7 Y	90700		LACERATION REPAIR, LAYERED	120--	
CONSULTATION/PRE-OP CLEARANCE				FLU, 6-35 MONTHS	90657		LESION, BIOPSY, ONE	11100	
EXPANDED PROBLEM FOCUSED	99242			FLU, 3Y+	90658		LESION, BIOPSY, EACH ADD'L	11101	
DETAILED	99243			HEP A, PED/ADOL, 2 DOSE	90633		LESION, DEST., BENIGN 1-14	17110	
COMPREHENSIVE/MOD COMPLEXITY	99244			HEP A, ADULT	90632		LESION DEST., PRE-MAL., SINGLE	17000	
COMPREHENSIVE/HIGH COMPLEXITY	99245			HEP B, PED/ADOL, 3 DOSE	90744		LESION DEST., PRE-MAL., EACH ADD'L	17003	
OTHER SERVICES				HEP B, ADULT	90746		LESION, EXCISION BENIGN	114--	
AFTER POSTED HOURS	99050			HEP B-HIB	90748		LESION, EXCISION, MALIGNANT	116--	
EVENING/WEEKEND APPT.	99051			HIB, 4 DOSE	90645		LESION, PARING/CUTTING, ONE	11055	
HOME HEALTH CERTIFICATION	G0180			HPV	90649		LESION PARING/CUTTING 2-4	11056	
HOME HEALTH RECERTIFICATION	G0179			IPV	90713		LESION, SHAVE	113--	
POST-OP FOLLOW UP	99024			MMR	90707		NAIL REMOVAL, PARTIAL	11730	
PROLONGED/30-74MIN	99354			PNEUMONIA, >2 Y	90732		NAIL REMOVAL, W/ MATRIX	11750	
SPECIAL REPORTS/FORMS	99080			PNEUMONIA CONJUGATE, <5Y	90669		SKIN TA, 1-15	11200	
DISABILITY/WORKERS COMP	99455			TD, > 7Y	90718		DENTAL (For practice purposes only)		
SPECIMIN HANDLING	99000			VARICELLA	90716		PERIODIC ORAL EVALUATION	DE0100	
OFFICE PROCEDURES				LABORATORY			COMPREHENSIVE EVALUATION	DE0150	
ANOSCOPY	46600			VENIPUNCTURE	36415		INTRAORAL, PERIAPICAL – 1ST FILM	DE0200	
AUDIOMETRY	92551			BLOOD GLUCOSE, MONITORING DEVICE	82962		INTRAORAL, PERIAPICAL–EACH ADD'L FILM	DE0250	
CERUMEN REMOVAL	69210			BLOOD GLUCOSE, VISUAL DIPSTICK	82948		BITEWING	DE026-	
COLPOSCOPY	54752			CBC, W/ AUTO DIFFERENTIAL	85025		PROPHYLAXIS - ADULT	DE1000	
COLPOSCOPY W/ BIOPSY	57455			CBC, W/O AUTO DIFFRENTIAL	85027		PROPHYLAXIS - CHILD	DE2000	
ECG W/ INTERPRETATION	93000			CHOLESTEROL	82465		PERIODONTAL MAINT.	DE5000	
ECG, RHYTHM STRIP	93040			HEMOOCULT, GUAIAC	82272		RESTORATIVE (ANTERIOR)	DE250-	
ENDOMETRIAL BIOPSY	58100			HEMOCCULT, IMMUNOASSAY	82274		RESTORATIVE (POSTERIOR)	DE260-	
FLEXIBLE SIGMOIDOSCOPY	45330			HEMOGLOBIN A1C	83036		FUSE CROWN-PORC	DE2700	
FLEXIBLE SIGMOIDOSCOPY W/ BIOPSY	45331			LIPID PANEL	80061		RE-CEMENT CROWN	DE2900	
FRACTURE CARE, CAST/SPLINT	29---			LIVER PANEL	80076		CORE BUILD UP INC. PINS	DE3000	
NEBULIZER	94640			KHO PREP (SKIN, HAIR, NAILS)	87220		CORE BUILD UP, PREFAB POST	DE3250	
NEBULIZER DEMO	94664			METABOLIC PANEL, BASIC	80048		LABIAL VENEER	DE3500	
SPIROMETRY	94010			METABOLIC PANEL, COMPHREHENSIVE	80053		CROWN - PORCELAIN FUSED TO GOLD	DE6000	
SPIROMETRY, PRE AND POST	94060			MONONUCLEOSIS	86663		CROWN LENGTHENING	DE4000	
TYMPANOMETRY	92567			PREGNANCY, BLOOD	84702		SURGICAL EXTRACTION	DE7000	
VASECTOMY	55250			PREGNANCY, URINE	81025		IMPACTED EXTRACTION	DE7250	
MEDICATIONS				RENAL PANEL	80069		LTD. ORTHO TREATMENT, ADULT	DE8000	
AMPICILIN, UP TO 500MG	J0290			SEDIMENTATION RATE	85652		ANALGESIA, NITROUS OXIDE	DE9000	

TODAY'S FEE		70.00
AMOUNT RECEIVED		35.00
BALANCE		35.00

WALDEN-MARTIN
FAMILY MEDICAL CLINIC
1234 ANYSTREET | ANYTOWN, ANYSTATE 12345
PHONE 123-123-1234 | FAX 123-123-5678

JULIE WALDEN MD
JAMES MARTIN MD
DAVID KAHN MD
ANGELA PEREZ MD
PATRICK TAYLOR DDS
JEAN BURKE NP

Patient Name: Willis, Erma
DOS: 11/13/2015
Diagnoses 1): L98.9
2): 702.11
3):
4):

SERVICE	CODE		PRICE	SERVICE	CODE	PRICE	SERVICE	CODE	PRICE
OFFICE VISIT	New	Est.		MEDICATIONS CONT'D			LABORATORY CONT'D		
MINIMAL OFFICE VISIT (OV)	99201	99211		B-12, UP TO 1,000MCG	J3420		STREP, RAPID	87880	
PROBLEM FOCUSED OV	99202	99212		EPINEPHINE, UP TO 1ML	J0170		STREP CULTURE	87081	
EXPANDED OV	99203	99213		KENALOG, 10MG	J3301		TB	87116	
DETAILED OV	99204	99214		LIDCAINE, 10MG	J2001		UA, COMPLETE, NON-AUTOMATED, MICRO	81000	
COMPHREHENSIVE OV	99205	99215		PROGESTERONE, 150MG	J1055		UA, W/O MICRO NON-AUTOMATED	81002	
WELLNESS VISIT	New	Est.		RECEPHIN, 250MG	J0696		UA, W/ MICRO, NON-AUTOMATED	81001	
WELL VISIT < 1 Y	99381	99391		TESTOSTERONE, 200MG	J1080		URINE COLONY COUNT	87086	
WELL VISIT 1-4 Y	99382	99392		TIGAN, UP TO 200MG	J3250		WET MOUNT/KOH	87210	
WELL VISIT 5-11 Y	99383	99393		TORADOL, 15MG	J1885		INPATIENT/OUTPATIENT PROCEDURES		
WELL VISIT 12-17 Y	99384	99394		NORMAL SALINE, 1000CC	J7030		UPPER GI ENDOSCOPY	43235	
WELL VISIT 18-39 Y	99385	99395		PHENERGAN, UP TO 50MG	J2550		UPPER GI ENDOSCOPY W/ BIOPSY	43239	
WELL VISIT 40-64 Y	99386	99396		IMMUNIZATIONS & INJECTIONS			UPPER GI ENDOSCOPY W/ GUIDE WIRE	43248	
WELL VISIT 65 Y+	99387	99397		ALLERGEN, ONE	95115		UPPER GI ENDOSCOPY W/ BALLOON	43249	
PREVENTATIVE SERVICES				ALLERGEN, MULTIPLE	95117		COLONOSCOPY	45378	
PAP	Q0091			IMM ADMIN, ONE	90471		COLONOSCOPY W/ BIOPSY	45380	
PELVIC & BREAST	G0101			IMM ADMIN, EACH ADD'L	90472		COLONOSCOPY W/ BIOPSY REMOVAL	45384	
PROSTATE/PSA	G0103			IMM ADMIN, INTRANASAL, ONE	90473		COLONOSCOPY W/ SNARE REMOVAL	45385	
TOBACCO COUNSELING/3-10MIN	99406			IMM ADMIN, INTRANASAL, EACH ADD'L	90475		SKIN PROCEDURES		
TOBACCO COUNSELING/>10MIN	99407			INJECTION, JOINT, SMALL	206--		BURN CARE, INITIAL	16000	
WELCOME TO MEDICARE EXAM	G0366			INJECTION, THER/PROPH/DIAG	90772		FROEIGN BODY, SKIN, SIMPLE	10120	
ECG W/ WELCOME TO MEDICARE EXAM	G0366			INJECTION, TRIGGER POINT	20552		FOREIGN BODY, SKIN, COMPLEX	12121	
FLEXIBLE SIGMOIDOSCOPY	G0104			VACCINES			I&D, ABSCESS	10060	
HEMOCCULT, GUAIAC	G0107			DT, <7 Y	90702		I&D, HEMATOMA/SEROMA	10140	
FLU ADMINISTRATION	G0008			DTP	90701		LCERATION REPAIR, SIMPLE	120--	
PENUMONIA ADMINISTRATION	G0009			DTAP, <7 Y	90700		LACERATION REPAIR, LAYERED	120--	
CONSULTATION/PRE-OP CLEARANCE				FLU, 6-35 MONTHS	90657		LESION, BIOPSY, ONE	11100	69.58
EXPANDED PROBLEM FOCUSED	99242			FLU, 3Y+	90658		LESION, BIOPSY, EACH ADD'L	11101	
DETAILED	99243			HEP A, PED/ADOL, 2 DOSE	90633		LESION, DEST., BENIGN 1-14	17110	38.00
COMPREHENSIVE/MOD COMPLEXITY	99244			HEP A, ADULT	90632		LESION DEST., PRE-MAL., SINGLE	17000	
COMPREHENSIVE/HIGH COMPLEXITY	99245			HEP B, PED/ADOL, 3 DOSE	90744		LESION DEST., PRE-MAL., EACH ADD'L	17003	
OTHER SERVICES				HEP B, ADULT	90746		LESION, EXCISION BENIGN	114--	
AFTER POSTED HOURS	99050			HEP B-HIB	90748		LESION, EXCISION, MALIGNANT	116--	
EVENING/WEEKEND APPT.	99051			HIB, 4 DOSE	90645		LESION, PARING/CUTTING, ONE	11055	
HOME HEALTH CERTIFICATION	G0180			HPV	90649		LESION PARING/CUTTING 2-4	11056	
HOME HEALTH RECERTIFICATION	G0179			IPV	90713		LESION, SHAVE	113--	
POST-OP FOLLOW UP	99024			MMR	90707		NAIL REMOVAL, PARTIAL	11730	
PROLONGED/30-74MIN	99354			PNEUMONIA, >2 Y	90732		NAIL REMOVAL, W/ MATRIX	11750	
SPECIAL REPORTS/FORMS	99080			PNEUMONIA CONJUGATE, <5Y	90669		SKIN TA, 1-15	11200	
DISABILITY/WORKERS COMP	99455			TD, > 7Y	90718		DENTAL (For practice purposes only)		
SPECIMIN HANDLING	99000			VARICELLA	90716		PERIODIC ORAL EVALUATION	DE0100	
OFFICE PROCEDURES				LABORATORY			COMPREHENSIVE EVALUATION	DE0150	
ANOSCOPY	46600			VENIPUNCTURE	36415		INTRAORAL, PERIAPICAL – 1ST FILM	DE0200	
AUDIOMETRY	92551			BLOOD GLUCOSE, MONITORING DEVICE	82962		INTRAORAL, PERIAPICAL–EACH ADD'L FILM	DE0250	
CERUMEN REMOVAL	69210			BLOOD GLUCOSE, VISUAL DIPSTICK	82948		BITEWING	DE026-	
COLPOSCOPY	54752			CBC, W/ AUTO DIFFERENTIAL	85025		PROPHYLAXIS - ADULT	DE1000	
COLPOSCOPY W/ BIOPSY	57455			CBC, W/O AUTO DIFFRENTIAL	85027		PROPHYLAXIS - CHILD	DE2000	
ECG W/ INTERPRETATION	93000			CHOLESTEROL	82465		PERIODONTAL MAINT.	DE5000	
ECG, RHYTHM STRIP	93040			HEMOOCULT, GUAIAC	82272		RESTORATIVE (ANTERIOR)	DE250-	
ENDOMETRIAL BIOPSY	58100			HEMOCCULT, IMMUNOASSAY	82274		RESTORATIVE (POSTERIOR)	DE260-	
FLEXIBLE SIGMOIDOSCOPY	45330			HEMOGLOBIN A1C	83036		FUSE CROWN-PORC	DE2700	
FLEXIBLE SIGMOIDOSCOPY W/ BIOPSY	45331			LIPID PANEL	80061		RE-CEMENT CROWN	DE2900	
FRACTURE CARE, CAST/SPLINT	29---			LIVER PANEL	80076		CORE BUILD UP INC. PINS	DE3000	
NEBULIZER	94640			KHO PREP (SKIN, HAIR, NAILS)	87220		CORE BUILD UP, PREFAB POST	DE3250	
NEBULIZER DEMO	94664			METABOLIC PANEL, BASIC	80048		LABIAL VENEER	DE3500	
SPIROMETRY	94010			METABOLIC PANEL, COMPHREHENSIVE	80053		CROWN - PORCELAIN FUSED TO GOLD	DE6000	
SPIROMETRY, PRE AND POST	94060			MONONUCLEOSIS	86663		CROWN LENGTHENING	DE4000	
TYMPANOMETRY	92567			PREGNANCY, BLOOD	84702		SURGICAL EXTRACTION	DE7000	
VASECTOMY	55250			PREGNANCY, URINE	81025		IMPACTED EXTRACTION	DE7250	
MEDICATIONS				RENAL PANEL	80069		LTD. ORTHO TREATMENT, ADULT	DE8000	
AMPICILIN, UP TO 500MG	J0290			SEDIMENTATION RATE	85652		ANALGESIA, NITROUS OXIDE	DE9000	

TODAY'S FEE		105.58
AMOUNT RECEIVED		0.00
BALANCE		105.58

Submitting a Medical Claim

Now that Norma Washington's superbill has been completed, it is time to submit a claim for her office visit. Remain in the Coding & Billing section of SimChart for the Medical Office and submit a claim for Norma's 8/14/2015 encounter and superbill.

Measurable Steps

1. Select Claim from the left Info Panel (Figure 3-9).

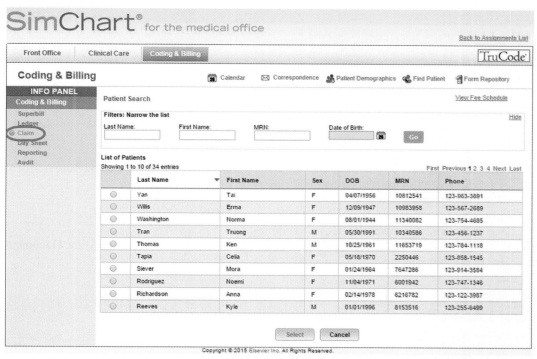

Figure 3-9 The Claim Option on the Left Info Panel.

2. Using the Patient Search field, search for Norma Washington's patient record.
3. Select the radio button for Norma Washington and click the select button.
4. Find the correct encounter and click on the edit tool (paper and pencil icon) next to it. Confirm the autopopulated details. Seven tabs appear within the claim: Patient Info, Provider Info, Payer Info, Encounter Notes, Claim Info, Charge Capture, and Submission (Figure 3-10). Certain patient demographic and encounter information is autopopulated in the claim.
5. Within the Patient Info tab, review the autopopulated information and document any additional information needed. Click the Save button.
6. Click the Provider Info tab and review the autopopulated information and document any additional information needed. Click the Save button.
7. Click the Payer Info tab and review the autopopulated information and document any additional information needed. Click the Save button.
8. Click the Encounter Notes tab.

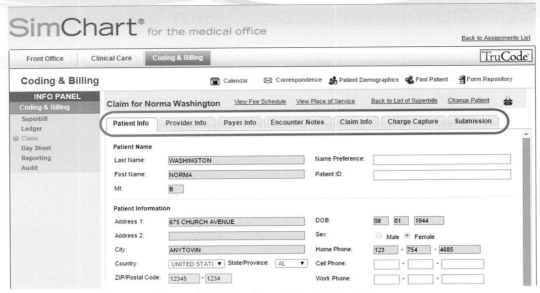

Figure 3-10 The Seven Tabs Within a Claim.

9. Select the Yes radio button to indicate that the HIPAA form is on file for Norma Washington and document the date of service in the Dated field.
10. Document any additional information needed and click the Save button.
11. Click the Claim Info tab and select the No radio buttons next to Employment and Auto Accident to indicate that this visit is not a claim on either and click the Save button.
12. Click the Charge Capture tab.
13. Document the encounter date in the DOS From and DOS To column.
14. Document "99213" in the CPT/HCPCS columns.
15. Use the View Place of Service link (Figure 3-11) to determine the correct POS code. Document "11" in the POS column.

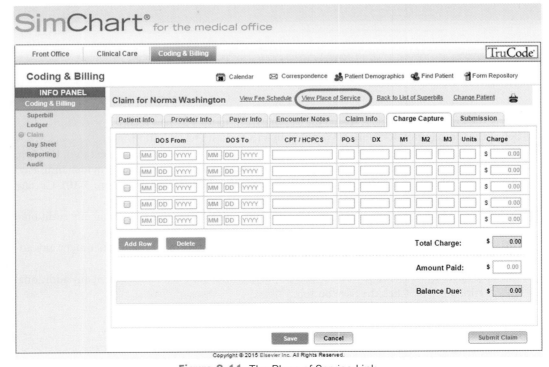

Figure 3-11 The Place of Service Link.

16. Document "1" in the DX column.

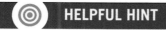
17. Document "1" in the Units column.
18. Document "43.00" in the Charge column.
19. Document any additional information needed and click the Save button.
20. Click on the Submission tab. Click in the "I am ready to submit the Claim" box.
21. Click on the Yes radio button to indicate that there is a signature on file and enter today's date in the Date field.
22. Click on the Submit Claim button. A confirmation message will appear (Figure 3-12).

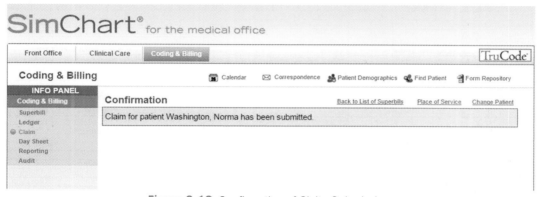

Figure 3-12 Confirmation of Claim Submission.

Submitting a Dental Claim

Reuven Ahmad was seen by Dr. Taylor for a filling on November 2, 2015. His superbill has already been completed in the system (Figure 3-13), but the claim needs to be submitted. Please complete and submit the claim for Reuven Ahmad.

WALDEN-MARTIN
FAMILY MEDICAL CLINIC
1234 ANYSTREET | ANYTOWN, ANYSTATE 12345
PHONE 123-123-1234 | FAX 123-123-5678

JULIE WALDEN MD
JAMES MARTIN MD
DAVID KAHN MD
ANGELA PEREZ MD
PATRICK TAYLOR DDS
JEAN BURKE NP

Patient Name: Ahmad, Reuven
DOS: 11/02/2015
Diagnoses 1):
2):
3):
4):

SERVICE	CODE		PRICE	SERVICE	CODE	PRICE	SERVICE	CODE	PRICE
OFFICE VISIT	New	Est.		MEDICATIONS CONT'D			LABORATORY CONT'D		
MINIMAL OFFICE VISIT (OV)	99201	99211		B-12, UP TO 1,000MCG	J3420		STREP, RAPID	87880	
PROBLEM FOCUSED OV	99202	99212		EPINEPHINE, UP TO 1ML	J0170		STREP CULTURE	87081	
EXPANDED OV	99203	99213		KENALOG, 10MG	J3301		TB	87116	
DETAILED OV	99204	99214		LIDCAINE, 10MG	J2001		UA, COMPLETE, NON-AUTOMATED, MICRO	81000	
COMPHREHENSIVE OV	99205	99215		PROGESTERONE, 150MG	J1055		UA, W/O MICRO NON-AUTOMATED	81002	
WELLNESS VISIT	New	Est.		RECEPHIN, 250MG	J0696		UA, W/ MICRO, NON-AUTOMATED	81001	
WELL VISIT <] Y	99381	99391		TESTOSTERONE, 200MG	J1080		URINE COLONY COUNT	87086	
WELL VISIT 1-4 Y	99382	99392		TIGAN, UP TO 200MG	J3250		WET MOUNT/KOH	87210	
WELL VISIT 5-11 Y	99383	99393		TORADOL, 15MG	J1885		INPATIENT/OUTPATIENT PROCEDURES		
WELL VISIT 12-17 Y	99384	99394		NORMAL SALINE, 1000CC	J7030		UPPER GI ENDOSCOPY	43235	
WELL VISIT 18-39 Y	99385	99395		PHENERGAN, UP TO 50MG	J2550		UPPER GI ENDOSCOPY W/ BIOPSY	43239	
WELL VISIT 40-64 Y	99386	99396		IMMUNIZATIONS & INJECTIONS			UPPER GI ENDOSCOPY W/ GUIDE WIRE	43248	
WELL VISIT 65 Y+	99387	99397		ALLERGEN, ONE	95115		UPPER GI ENDOSCOPY W/ BALLOON	43249	
PREVENTATIVE SERVICES				ALLERGEN, MULTIPLE	95117		COLONOSCOPY	45378	
PAP	Q0091			IMM ADMIN, ONE	90471		COLONOSCOPY W/ BIOPSY	45380	
PELVIC & BREAST	G0101			IMM ADMIN, EACH ADD'L	90472		COLONOSCOPY W/ BIOPSY REMOVAL	45384	
PROSTATE/PSA	G0103			IMM ADMIN, INTRANASAL, ONE	90473		COLONOSCOPY W/ SNARE REMOVAL	45385	
TOBACCO COUNSELING/3-10MIN	99406			IMM ADMIN, INTRANASAL, EACH ADD'L	90475		SKIN PROCEDURES		
TOBACCO COUNSELING/>10MIN	99407			INJECTION, JOINT, SMALL	206--		BURN CARE, INITIAL	16000	
WELCOME TO MEDICARE EXAM	G0366			INJECTION, THER/PROPH/DIAG	90772		FROEIGN BODY, SKIN, SIMPLE	10120	
ECG W/ WELCOME TO MEDICARE EXAM	G0366			INJECTION, TRIGGER POINT	20552		FOREIGN BODY, SKIN, COMPLEX	12121	
FLEXIBLE SIGMOIDOSCOPY	G0104			VACCINES			I&D, ABSCESS	10060	
HEMOCCULT, GUAIAC	G0107			DT, <7 Y	90702		I&D, HEMATOMA/SEROMA	10140	
FLU ADMINISTRATION	G0008			DTP	90701		LCERATION REPAIR, SIMPLE	120--	
PENUMONIA ADMINISTRATION	G0009			DTAP, <7 Y	90700		LACERATION REPAIR, LAYERED	120--	
CONSULTATION/PRE-OP CLEARANCE				FLU, 6-35 MONTHS	90657		LESION, BIOPSY, ONE	11100	
EXPANDED PROBLEM FOCUSED	99242			FLU, 3Y+	90658		LESION, BIOPSY, EACH ADD'L	11101	
DETAILED	99243			HEP A, PED/ADOL, 2 DOSE	90633		LESION, DEST., BENIGN 1-14	17110	
COMPREHENSIVE/MOD COMPLEXITY	99244			HEP A, ADULT	90632		LESION DEST., PRE-MAL., SINGLE	17000	
COMPREHENSIVE/HIGH COMPLEXITY	99245			HEP B, PED/ADOL, 3 DOSE	90744		LESION DEST., PRE-MAL., EACH ADD'L	17003	
OTHER SERVICES				HEP B, ADULT	90746		LESION, EXCISION BENIGN	114--	
AFTER POSTED HOURS	99050			HEP B-HIB	90748		LESION, EXCISION, MALIGNANT	116--	
EVENING/WEEKEND APPT.	99051			HIB, 4 DOSE	90645		LESION, PARING/CUTTING, ONE	11055	
HOME HEALTH CERTIFICATION	G0180			HPV	90649		LESION PARING/CUTTING 2-4	11056	
HOME HEALTH RECERTIFICATION	G0179			IPV	90713		LESION, SHAVE	113--	
POST-OP FOLLOW UP	99024			MMR	90707		NAIL REMOVAL, PARTIAL	11730	
PROLONGED/30-74MIN	99354			PNEUMONIA, >2 Y	90732		NAIL REMOVAL, W/ MATRIX	11750	
SPECIAL REPORTS/FORMS	99080			PNEUMONIA CONJUGATE, <5Y	90669		SKIN TA, 1-15	11200	
DISABILITY/WORKERS COMP	99455			TD, > 7Y	90718		DENTAL (For practice purposes only)		
SPECIMIN HANDLING	99000			VARICELLA	90716		PERIODIC ORAL EVALUATION	DE0100	
OFFICE PROCEDURES				LABORATORY			COMPREHENSIVE EVALUATION	DE0150	
ANOSCOPY	46600			VENIPUNCTURE	36415		INTRAORAL, PERIAPICAL – 1ST FILM	DE0200	
AUDIOMETRY	92551			BLOOD GLUCOSE, MONITORING DEVICE	82962		INTRAORAL, PERIAPICAL--EACH ADD'L FILM	DE0250	
CERUMEN REMOVAL	69210			BLOOD GLUCOSE, VISUAL DIPSTICK	82948		BITEWING	DE026-	
COLPOSCOPY	54752			CBC, W/ AUTO DIFFERENTIAL	85025		PROPHYLAXIS - ADULT	DE1000	
COLPOSCOPY W/ BIOPSY	57455			CBC, W/O AUTO DIFFRENTIAL	85027		PROPHYLAXIS - CHILD	DE2000	
ECG W/ INTERPRETATION	93000			CHOLESTEROL	82465		PERIODONTAL MAINT.	DE5000	
ECG, RHYTHM STRIP	93040			HEMOCCULT, GUAIAC	82272		RESTORATIVE (ANTERIOR)	DE250-	
ENDOMETRIAL BIOPSY	58100			HEMOCCULT, IMMUNOASSAY	82274		RESTORATIVE (POSTERIOR)	DE2603	242.00
FLEXIBLE SIGMOIDOSCOPY	45330			HEMOGLOBIN A1C	83036		FUSE CROWN-PORC	DE2700	
FLEXIBLE SIGMOIDOSCOPY W/ BIOPSY	45331			LIPID PANEL	80061		RE-CEMENT CROWN	DE2900	
FRACTURE CARE, CAST/SPLINT	29---			LIVER PANEL	80076		CORE BUILD UP INC. PINS	DE3000	
NEBULIZER	94640			KHO PREP (SKIN, HAIR, NAILS)	87220		CORE BUILD UP, PREFAB POST	DE3250	
NEBULIZER DEMO	94664			METABOLIC PANEL, BASIC	80048		LABIAL VENEER	DE3500	
SPIROMETRY	94010			METABOLIC PANEL, COMPHREHENSIVE	80053		CROWN - PORCELAIN FUSED TO GOLD	DE6000	
SPIROMETRY, PRE AND POST	94060			MONONUCLEOSIS	86663		CROWN LENGTHENING	DE4000	
TYMPANOMETRY	92567			PREGNANCY, BLOOD	84702		SURGICAL EXTRACTION	DE7000	
VASECTOMY	55250			PREGNANCY, URINE	81025		IMPACTED EXTRACTION	DE7250	
MEDICATIONS				RENAL PANEL	80069		LTD. ORTHO TREATMENT, ADULT	DE8000	
AMPICILIN, UP TO 500MG	J0290			SEDIMENTATION RATE	85652		ANALGESIA, NITROUS OXIDE	DE9000	

TODAY'S FEE		242.00
AMOUNT RECEIVED		0.00
BALANCE		242.00

Figure 3-13 Dental Superbill for Reuven Ahmad.

HELPFUL HINT

A dental claim is nearly identical to a medical claim, with the main difference being in the Charge Capture tab. Currently diagnosis codes are not required for dental claims, but dentists must provide information on specific teeth and surfaces that are treated.

Measurable Steps

1. Select Claim from the left Info Panel.
2. Using the Patient Search field, search for Reuven Ahmad's patient record.
3. Select the radio button for Reuven Ahmad and click the select button.
4. Find the correct encounter and click on the edit tool (paper and pencil icon) next to it. Confirm the autopopulated details.
5. Within the Patient Info tab, review the autopopulated information and document any additional information needed. Click the Save button.
6. Click the Provider Info tab and review the autopopulated information and document any additional information needed. Click the Save button.
7. Click the Payer Info tab and review the autopopulated information and document any additional information needed. Click the Save button.
8. Click the Encounter Notes tab.
9. Select the Yes radio button to indicate that the HIPAA form is on file for Reuven Ahmad and document the date of service in the Dated field.
10. Document any additional information needed and click the Save button.
11. Click the Claim Info tab and select the No radio buttons next to Employment and Auto Accident to indicate that this visit is not a claim on either and click the Save button.
12. Click the Charge Capture tab.
13. Document the encounter date in the DOS From and DOS To column.
14. Document the code "D2393" in the CPT/HCPCS Column.
15. Document "11" in the POS column.
16. Leave the DX, Area of Cavity, and Tooth System columns blank.

HELPFUL HINT

Remember that diagnosis codes are not mandatory on dental claims.

17. Document "4" in the Tooth # column.
18. Document "MOD" in the Surface column.
19. Document "1" in the Units column.
20. Document "242.00" in the Charge column.
21. Document any additional information needed and click the Save button.
22. Click on the Submission tab. Click in the "I am ready to submit the Claim" box.
23. Click on the Yes radio button to indicate that there is a signature on file and enter today's date in the Date field.
24. Click on the Submit Claim button. A confirmation message will appear.

WALDEN-MARTIN
FAMILY MEDICAL CLINIC
1234 ANYSTREET | ANYTOWN, ANYSTATE 12345
PHONE 123-123-1234 | FAX 123-123-5678

JULIE WALDEN MD
JAMES MARTIN MD
DAVID KAHN MD
ANGELA PEREZ MD
(PATRICK TAYLOR DDS)
JEAN BURKE NP

Patient Name: Ahmad, Reuven
DOS: 11/02/2015
Diagnoses 1):
2):
3):
4):

SERVICE	CODE New	Est.	PRICE	SERVICE	CODE	PRICE	SERVICE	CODE	PRICE
OFFICE VISIT				MEDICATIONS CONT'D			LABORATORY CONT'D		
MINIMAL OFFICE VISIT (OV)	99201	99211		B-12, UP TO 1,000MCG	J3420		STREP, RAPID	87880	
PROBLEM FOCUSED OV	99202	99212		EPINEPHINE, UP TO 1ML	J0170		STREP CULTURE	87081	
EXPANDED OV	99203	99213		KENALOG, 10MG	J3301		TB	87116	
DETAILED OV	99204	99214		LIDCAINE, 10MG	J2001		UA, COMPLETE, NON-AUTOMATED, MICRO	81000	
COMPHREHENSIVE OV	99205	99215		PROGESTERONE, 150MG	J1055		UA, W/O MICRO NON-AUTOMATED	81002	
WELLNESS VISIT	New	Est.		RECEPHIN, 250MG	J0696		UA, W/ MICRO, NON-AUTOMATED	81001	
WELL VISIT < 1 Y	99381	99391		TESTOSTERONE, 200MG	J1080		URINE COLONY COUNT	87086	
WELL VISIT 1-4 Y	99382	99392		TIGAN, UP TO 200MG	J3250		WET MOUNT/KOH	87210	
WELL VISIT 5-11 Y	99383	99393		TORADOL, 15MG	J1885		INPATIENT/OUTPATIENT PROCEDURES		
WELL VISIT 12-17 Y	99384	99394		NORMAL SALINE, 1000CC	J7030		UPPER GI ENDOSCOPY	43235	
WELL VISIT 18-39 Y	99385	99395		PHENERGAN, UP TO 50MG	J2550		UPPER GI ENDOSCOPY W/ BIOPSY	43239	
WELL VISIT 40-64 Y	99386	99396		IMMUNIZATIONS & INJECTIONS			UPPER GI ENDOSCOPY W/ GUIDE WIRE	43248	
WELL VISIT 65 Y+	99387	99397		ALLERGEN, ONE	95115		UPPER GI ENDOSCOPY W/ BALLOON	43249	
PREVENTATIVE SERVICES				ALLERGEN, MULTIPLE	95117		COLONOSCOPY	45378	
PAP	Q0091			IMM ADMIN, ONE	90471		COLONOSCOPY W/ BIOPSY	45380	
PELVIC & BREAST	G0101			IMM ADMIN, EACH ADD'L	90472		COLONOSCOPY W/ BIOPSY REMOVAL	45384	
PROSTATE/PSA	G0103			IMM ADMIN, INTRANASAL, ONE	90473		COLONOSCOPY W/ SNARE REMOVAL	45385	
TOBACCO COUNSELING/3-10MIN	99406			IMM ADMIN, INTRANASAL, EACH ADD'L	90475		SKIN PROCEDURES		
TOBACCO COUNSELING/>10MIN	99407			INJECTION, JOINT, SMALL	206--		BURN CARE, INITIAL	16000	
WELCOME TO MEDICARE EXAM	G0366			INJECTION, THER/PROPH/DIAG	90772		FROEIGN BODY, SKIN, SIMPLE	10120	
ECG W/ WELCOME TO MEDICARE EXAM	G0366			INJECTION, TRIGGER POINT	20552		FOREIGN BODY, SKIN, COMPLEX	12121	
FLEXIBLE SIGMOIDOSCOPY	G0104			VACCINES			I&D, ABSCESS	10060	
HEMOCCULT, GUAIAC	G0107			DT, <7 Y	90702		I&D, HEMATOMA/SEROMA	10140	
FLU ADMINISTRATION	G0008			DTP	90701		LCERATION REPAIR, SIMPLE	120--	
PENUMONIA ADMINISTRATION	G0009			DTAP, <7 Y	90700		LACERATION REPAIR, LAYERED	120--	
CONSULTATION/PRE-OP CLEARANCE				FLU, 6-35 MONTHS	90657		LESION, BIOPSY, ONE	11100	
EXPANDED PROBLEM FOCUSED	99242			FLU, 3Y+	90658		LESION, BIOPSY, EACH ADD'L	11101	
DETAILED	99243			HEP A, PED/ADOL, 2 DOSE	90633		LESION, DEST., BENIGN 1-14	17110	
COMPREHENSIVE/MOD COMPLEXITY	99244			HEP A, ADULT	90632		LESION DEST., PRE-MAL., SINGLE	17000	
COMPREHENSIVE/HIGH COMPLEXITY	99245			HEP B, PED/ADOL, 3 DOSE	90744		LESION DEST., PRE-MAL., EACH ADD'L	17003	
OTHER SERVICES				HEP B, ADULT	90746		LESION, EXCISION BENIGN	114--	
AFTER POSTED HOURS	99050			HEP B-HIB	90748		LESION, EXCISION, MALIGNANT	116--	
EVENING/WEEKEND APPT.	99051			HIB, 4 DOSE	90645		LESION, PARING/CUTTING, ONE	11055	
HOME HEALTH CERTIFICATION	G0180			HPV	90649		LESION PARING/CUTTING 2-4	11056	
HOME HEALTH RECERTIFICATION	G0179			IPV	90713		LESION, SHAVE	113--	
POST-OP FOLLOW UP	99024			MMR	90707		NAIL REMOVAL, PARTIAL	11730	
PROLONGED/30-74MIN	99354			PNEUMONIA, >2 Y	90732		NAIL REMOVAL, W/ MATRIX	11750	
SPECIAL REPORTS/FORMS	99080			PNEUMONIA CONJUGATE, <5Y	90669		SKIN TA, 1-15	11200	
DISABILITY/WORKERS COMP	99455			TD, > 7Y	90718		DENTAL (For practice purposes only)		
SPECIMIN HANDLING	99000			VARICELLA	90716		PERIODIC ORAL EVALUATION	DE0100	
OFFICE PROCEDURES				LABORATORY			COMPREHENSIVE EVALUATION	DE0150	
ANOSCOPY	46600			VENIPUNCTURE	36415		INTRAORAL, PERIAPICAL – 1ST FILM	DE0200	
AUDIOMETRY	92551			BLOOD GLUCOSE, MONITORING DEVICE	82962		INTRAORAL, PERIAPICAL–EACH ADD'L FILM	DE0250	
CERUMEN REMOVAL	69210			BLOOD GLUCOSE, VISUAL DIPSTICK	82948		BITEWING	DE026-	
COLPOSCOPY	54752			CBC, W/ AUTO DIFFERENTIAL	85025		PROPHYLAXIS - ADULT	DE1000	
COLPOSCOPY W/ BIOPSY	57455			CBC, W/O AUTO DIFFRENTIAL	85027		PROPHYLAXIS - CHILD	DE2000	
ECG W/ INTERPRETATION	93000			CHOLESTEROL	82465		PERIODONTAL MAINT.	DE5000	
ECG, RHYTHM STRIP	93040			HEMOOCULT, GUAIAC	82272		RESTORATIVE (ANTERIOR)	DE250-	
ENDOMETRIAL BIOPSY	58100			HEMOCCULT, IMMUNOASSAY	82274		RESTORATIVE (POSTERIOR)	DE2603	242.00
FLEXIBLE SIGMOIDOSCOPY	45330			HEMOGLOBIN A1C	83036		FUSE CROWN-PORC	DE2700	
FLEXIBLE SIGMOIDOSCOPY W/ BIOPSY	45331			LIPID PANEL	80061		RE-CEMENT CROWN	DE2900	
FRACTURE CARE, CAST/SPLINT	29---			LIVER PANEL	80076		CORE BUILD UP INC. PINS	DE3000	
NEBULIZER	94640			KHO PREP (SKIN, HAIR, NAILS)	87220		CORE BUILD UP, PREFAB POST	DE3250	
NEBULIZER DEMO	94664			METABOLIC PANEL, BASIC	80048		LABIAL VENEER	DE3500	
SPIROMETRY	94010			METABOLIC PANEL, COMPHREHENSIVE	80053		CROWN - PORCELAIN FUSED TO GOLD	DE6000	
SPIROMETRY, PRE AND POST	94060			MONONUCLEOSIS	86663		CROWN LENGTHENING	DE4000	
TYMPANOMETRY	92567			PREGNANCY, BLOOD	84702		SURGICAL EXTRACTION	DE7000	
VASECTOMY	55250			PREGNANCY, URINE	81025		IMPACTED EXTRACTION	DE7250	
MEDICATIONS				RENAL PANEL	80069		LTD. ORTHO TREATMENT, ADULT	DE8000	
AMPICILIN, UP TO 500MG	J0290			SEDIMENTATION RATE	85652		ANALGESIA, NITROUS OXIDE	DE9000	

TODAY'S FEE		242.00
AMOUNT RECEIVED		0.00
BALANCE		242.00

WALDEN-MARTIN
FAMILY MEDICAL CLINIC
1234 ANYSTREET | ANYTOWN, ANYSTATE 12345
PHONE 123-123-1234 | FAX 123-123-5678

JULIE WALDEN MD
JAMES MARTIN MD
DAVID KAHN MD
ANGELA PEREZ MD
PATRICK TAYLOR DDS
JEAN BURKE NP

PATIENT INFO

First Name		MI	Last Name		Date of Birth		Sex

SSN		Preferred Phone		Dental Insurance		Responsible Party

BRIEF HISTORY

Last Visit	Treatment		X-Rays: Y / N

CLINICAL DATA

General Condition of Teeth

General Condition of Gums

General Condition of the Floor of the Mouth

Examination and treatment plan—List in order from tooth no. 1 through no. 32—Use charting system shown

Identify missing teeth with "x"

Upper

Right

Left

Primary   Permanent

Lower

Tooth # or letter	Surface	Description of service (including x-ray, prophylaxis, materials used, etc.)	Date service performed Mo./Day/Year	Procedure number

Remarks for unusual services

Follow up:

Activity

Now submit claims for all of the superbills generated in the first Activity of this unit (pp. 55-65). Additionally, you will submit claims for two superbills that have already been completed in the system. See the following two hard copies to assist you with entering the correct information.

HELPFUL HINT

If a patient is self-pay, you will not submit a claim to an insurance provider. The patient will be billed later. Please skip this activity for any self-pay patients.

WALDEN-MARTIN
FAMILY MEDICAL CLINIC
1234 ANYSTREET | ANYTOWN, ANYSTATE 12345
PHONE 123-123-1234 | FAX 123-123-5678

JULIE WALDEN MD
JAMES MARTIN MD
DAVID KAHN MD
ANGELA PEREZ MD
PATRICK TAYLOR DDS
JEAN BURKE NP

Patient Name: Nasser, Talibah
DOS: 10/28/15
Diagnoses 1): J11.1
2):
3):
4):

SERVICE	CODE New	Est.	PRICE	SERVICE	CODE	PRICE	SERVICE	CODE	PRICE
OFFICE VISIT	New	Est.		MEDICATIONS CONT'D			LABORATORY CONT'D		
MINIMAL OFFICE VISIT (OV)	99201	99211		B-12, UP TO 1,000MCG	J3420		STREP, RAPID	87880	
PROBLEM FOCUSED OV	99202	99212	32.00	EPINEPHINE, UP TO 1ML	J0170		STREP CULTURE	87081	
EXPANDED OV	99203	99213		KENALOG, 10MG	J3301		TB	87116	
DETAILED OV	99204	99214		LIDCAINE, 10MG	J2001		UA, COMPLETE, NON-AUTOMATED, MICRO	81000	
COMPHREHENSIVE OV	99205	99215		PROGESTERONE, 150MG	J1055		UA, W/O MICRO NON-AUTOMATED	81002	
WELLNESS VISIT	New	Est.		RECEPHIN, 250MG	J0696		UA, W/ MICRO, NON-AUTOMATED	81001	
WELL VISIT < 1 Y	99381	99391		TESTOSTERONE, 200MG	J1080		URINE COLONY COUNT	87086	
WELL VISIT 1-4 Y	99382	99392		TIGAN, UP TO 200MG	J3250		WET MOUNT/KOH	87210	
WELL VISIT 5-11 Y	99383	99393		TORADOL, 15MG	J1885		INPATIENT/OUTPATIENT PROCEDURES		
WELL VISIT 12-17 Y	99384	99394		NORMAL SALINE, 1000CC	J7030		UPPER GI ENDOSCOPY	43235	
WELL VISIT 18-39 Y	99385	99395		PHENERGAN, UP TO 50MG	J2550		UPPER GI ENDOSCOPY W/ BIOPSY	43239	
WELL VISIT 40-64 Y	99386	99396		IMMUNIZATIONS & INJECTIONS			UPPER GI ENDOSCOPY W/ GUIDE WIRE	43248	
WELL VISIT 65 Y+	99387	99397		ALLERGEN, ONE	95115		UPPER GI ENDOSCOPY W/ BALLOON	43249	
PREVENTATIVE SERVICES				ALLERGEN, MULTIPLE	95117		COLONOSCOPY	45378	
PAP	Q0091			IMM ADMIN, ONE	90471		COLONOSCOPY W/ BIOPSY	45380	
PELVIC & BREAST	G0101			IMM ADMIN, EACH ADD'L	90472		COLONOSCOPY W/ BIOPSY REMOVAL	45384	
PROSTATE/PSA	G0103			IMM ADMIN, INTRANASAL, ONE	90473		COLONOSCOPY W/ SNARE REMOVAL	45385	
TOBACCO COUNSELING/3-10MIN	99406			IMM ADMIN, INTRANASAL, EACH ADD'L	90475		SKIN PROCEDURES		
TOBACCO COUNSELING/>10MIN	99407			INJECTION, JOINT, SMALL	206--		BURN CARE, INITIAL	16000	
WELCOME TO MEDICARE EXAM	G0366			INJECTION, THER/PROPH/DIAG	90772		FROEIGN BODY, SKIN, SIMPLE	10120	
ECG W/ WELCOME TO MEDICARE EXAM	G0366			INJECTION, TRIGGER POINT	20552		FOREIGN BODY, SKIN, COMPLEX	12121	
FLEXIBLE SIGMOIDOSCOPY	G0104			VACCINES			I&D, ABSCESS	10060	
HEMOCCULT, GUAIAC	G0107			DT, <7 Y	90702		I&D, HEMATOMA/SEROMA	10140	
FLU ADMINISTRATION	G0008			DTP	90701		LCERATION REPAIR, SIMPLE	120--	
PENUMONIA ADMINISTRATION	G0009			DTAP, <7 Y	90700		LACERATION REPAIR, LAYERED	120--	
CONSULTATION/PRE-OP CLEARANCE				FLU, 6-35 MONTHS	90657		LESION, BIOPSY, ONE	11100	
EXPANDED PROBLEM FOCUSED	99242			FLU, 3Y+	90658		LESION, BIOPSY, EACH ADD'L	11101	
DETAILED	99243			HEP A, PED/ADOL, 2 DOSE	90633		LESION, DEST., BENIGN 1-14	17110	
COMPREHENSIVE/MOD COMPLEXITY	99244			HEP A, ADULT	90632		LESION DEST., PRE-MAL., SINGLE	17000	
COMPREHENSIVE/HIGH COMPLEXITY	99245			HEP B, PED/ADOL, 3 DOSE	90744		LESION DEST., PRE-MAL., EACH ADD'L	17003	
OTHER SERVICES				HEP B, ADULT	90746		LESION, EXCISION BENIGN	114--	
AFTER POSTED HOURS	99050			HEP B-HIB	90748		LESION, EXCISION, MALIGNANT	116--	
EVENING/WEEKEND APPT.	99051			HIB, 4 DOSE	90645		LESION, PARING/CUTTING, ONE	11055	
HOME HEALTH CERTIFICATION	G0180			HPV	90649		LESION PARING/CUTTING 2-4	11056	
HOME HEALTH RECERTIFICATION	G0179			IPV	90713		LESION, SHAVE	113--	
POST-OP FOLLOW UP	99024			MMR	90707		NAIL REMOVAL, PARTIAL	11730	
PROLONGED/30-74MIN	99354			PNEUMONIA, >2 Y	90732		NAIL REMOVAL, W/ MATRIX	11750	
SPECIAL REPORTS/FORMS	99080			PNEUMONIA CONJUGATE, <5Y	90669		SKIN TA, 1-15	11200	
DISABILITY/WORKERS COMP	99455			TD, > 7Y	90718		DENTAL (For practice purposes only)		
SPECIMIN HANDLING	99000			VARICELLA	90716		PERIODIC ORAL EVALUATION	DE0100	
OFFICE PROCEDURES				LABORATORY			COMPREHENSIVE EVALUATION	DE0150	
ANOSCOPY	46600			VENIPUNCTURE	36415		INTRAORAL, PERIAPICAL – 1ST FILM	DE0200	
AUDIOMETRY	92551			BLOOD GLUCOSE, MONITORING DEVICE	82962		INTRAORAL, PERIAPICAL–EACH ADD'L FILM	DE0250	
CERUMEN REMOVAL	69210			BLOOD GLUCOSE, VISUAL DIPSTICK	82948		BITEWING	DE026-	
COLPOSCOPY	54752			CBC, W/ AUTO DIFFERENTIAL	85025		PROPHYLAXIS - ADULT	DE1000	
COLPOSCOPY W/ BIOPSY	57455			CBC, W/O AUTO DIFFERENTIAL	85027		PROPHYLAXIS - CHILD	DE2000	
ECG W/ INTERPRETATION	93000			CHOLESTEROL	82465		PERIODONTAL MAINT.	DE5000	
ECG, RHYTHM STRIP	93040			HEMOOCULT, GUAIAC	82272		RESTORATIVE (ANTERIOR)	DE250-	
ENDOMETRIAL BIOPSY	58100			HEMOCCULT, IMMUNOASSAY	82274		RESTORATIVE (POSTERIOR)	DE260-	
FLEXIBLE SIGMOIDOSCOPY	45330			HEMOGLOBIN A1C	83036		FUSE CROWN-PORC	DE2700	
FLEXIBLE SIGMOIDOSCOPY W/ BIOPSY	45331			LIPID PANEL	80061		RE-CEMENT CROWN	DE2900	
FRACTURE CARE, CAST/SPLINT	29---			LIVER PANEL	80076		CORE BUILD UP INC. PINS	DE3000	
NEBULIZER	94640			KHO PREP (SKIN, HAIR, NAILS)	87220		CORE BUILD UP, PREFAB POST	DE3250	
NEBULIZER DEMO	94664			METABOLIC PANEL, BASIC	80048		LABIAL VENEER	DE3500	
SPIROMETRY	94010			METABOLIC PANEL, COMPHREHENSIVE	80053		CROWN - PORCELAIN FUSED TO GOLD	DE6000	
SPIROMETRY, PRE AND POST	94060			MONONUCLEOSIS	86663		CROWN LENGTHENING	DE4000	
TYMPANOMETRY	92567			PREGNANCY, BLOOD	84702		SURGICAL EXTRACTION	DE7000	
VASECTOMY	55250			PREGNANCY, URINE	81025		IMPACTED EXTRACTION	DE7250	
MEDICATIONS				RENAL PANEL	80069		LTD. ORTHO TREATMENT, ADULT	DE8000	
AMPICILIN, UP TO 500MG	J0290			SEDIMENTATION RATE	85652		ANALGESIA, NITROUS OXIDE	DE9000	

TODAY'S FEE		32.00
AMOUNT RECEIVED		25.00
BALANCE		7.00

WALDEN-MARTIN
FAMILY MEDICAL CLINIC
1234 ANYSTREET | ANYTOWN, ANYSTATE 12345
PHONE 123-123-1234 | FAX 123-123-5678

JULIE WALDEN MD
JAMES MARTIN MD
DAVID KAHN MD
ANGELA PEREZ MD
PATRICK TAYLOR DDS
(JEAN BURKE NP)

Patient Name: Parker, Johnny
DOS: 10/30/15
Diagnoses 1): Z00.129
2):
3):
4):

SERVICE	CODE		PRICE	SERVICE	CODE	PRICE	SERVICE	CODE	PRICE
OFFICE VISIT	New	Est.		**MEDICATIONS CONT'D**			**LABORATORY CONT'D**		
MINIMAL OFFICE VISIT (OV)	99201	99211		B-12, UP TO 1,000MCG	J3420		STREP, RAPID	87880	
PROBLEM FOCUSED OV	99202	99212		EPINEPHINE, UP TO 1ML	J0170		STREP CULTURE	87081	
EXPANDED OV	99203	99213		KENALOG, 10MG	J3301		TB	87116	
DETAILED OV	99204	99214		LIDCAINE, 10MG	J2001		UA, COMPLETE, NON-AUTOMATED, MICRO	81000	
COMPHREHENSIVE OV	99205	99215		PROGESTERONE, 150MG	J1055		UA, W/O MICRO NON-AUTOMATED	81002	
WELLNESS VISIT	New	Est.		RECEPHIN, 250MG	J0696		UA, W/ MICRO, NON-AUTOMATED	81001	
WELL VISIT < 1 Y	99381	99391		TESTOSTERONE, 200MG	J1080		URINE COLONY COUNT	87086	
WELL VISIT 1-4 Y	99382	99392	75.00	TIGAN, UP TO 200MG	J3250		WET MOUNT/KOH	87210	
WELL VISIT 5-11 Y	99383	99393		TORADOL, 15MG	J1885		**INPATIENT/OUTPATIENT PROCEDURES**		
WELL VISIT 12-17 Y	99384	99394		NORMAL SALINE, 1000CC	J7030		UPPER GI ENDOSCOPY	43235	
WELL VISIT 18-39 Y	99385	99395		PHENERGAN, UP TO 50MG	J2550		UPPER GI ENDOSCOPY W/ BIOPSY	43239	
WELL VISIT 40-64 Y	99386	99396		**IMMUNIZATIONS & INJECTIONS**			UPPER GI ENDOSCOPY W/ GUIDE WIRE	43248	
WELL VISIT 65 Y+	99387	99397		ALLERGEN, ONE	95115		UPPER GI ENDOSCOPY W/ BALLOON	43249	
PREVENTATIVE SERVICES				ALLERGEN, MULTIPLE	95117		COLONOSCOPY	45378	
PAP	Q0091			IMM ADMIN, ONE	90471		COLONOSCOPY W/ BIOPSY	45380	
PELVIC & BREAST	G0101			IMM ADMIN, EACH ADD'L	90472		COLONOSCOPY W/ BIOPSY REMOVAL	45384	
PROSTATE/PSA	G0103			IMM ADMIN, INTRANASAL, ONE	90473		COLONOSCOPY W/ SNARE REMOVAL	45385	
TOBACCO COUNSELING/3-10MIN	99406			IMM ADMIN, INTRANASAL, EACH ADD'L	90475		**SKIN PROCEDURES**		
TOBACCO COUNSELING/>10MIN	99407			INJECTION, JOINT, SMALL	206--		BURN CARE, INITIAL	16000	
WELCOME TO MEDICARE EXAM	G0366			INJECTION, THER/PROPH/DIAG	90772		FROEIGN BODY, SKIN, SIMPLE	10120	
ECG W/ WELCOME TO MEDICARE EXAM	G0366			INJECTION, TRIGGER POINT	20552		FOREIGN BODY, SKIN, COMPLEX	12121	
FLEXIBLE SIGMOIDOSCOPY	G0104			**VACCINES**			I&D, ABSCESS	10060	
HEMOCCULT, GUAIAC	G0107			DT, <7 Y	90702		I&D, HEMATOMA/SEROMA	10140	
FLU ADMINISTRATION	G0008			DTP	90701		LCERATION REPAIR, SIMPLE	120--	
PENUMONIA ADMINISTRATION	G0009			DTAP, <7 Y	90700		LACERATION REPAIR, LAYERED	120--	
CONSULTATION/PRE-OP CLEARANCE				FLU, 6-35 MONTHS	90657		LESION, BIOPSY, ONE	11100	
EXPANDED PROBLEM FOCUSED	99242			FLU, 3Y+	90658		LESION, BIOPSY, EACH ADD'L	11101	
DETAILED	99243			HEP A, PED/ADOL, 2 DOSE	90633		LESION, DEST., BENIGN 1-14	17110	
COMPREHENSIVE/MOD COMPLEXITY	99244			HEP A, ADULT	90632		LESION DEST., PRE-MAL., SINGLE	17000	
COMPREHENSIVE/HIGH COMPLEXITY	99245			HEP B, PED/ADOL, 3 DOSE	90744		LESION DEST., PRE-MAL., EACH ADD'L	17003	
OTHER SERVICES				HEP B, ADULT	90746		LESION, EXCISION BENIGN	114--	
AFTER POSTED HOURS	99050			HEP B-HIB	90748		LESION, EXCISION, MALIGNANT	116--	
EVENING/WEEKEND APPT.	99051			HIB, 4 DOSE	90645		LESION, PARING/CUTTING, ONE	11055	
HOME HEALTH CERTIFICATION	G0180			HPV	90649		LESION PARING/CUTTING 2-4	11056	
HOME HEALTH RECERTIFICATION	G0179			IPV	90713		LESION, SHAVE	113--	
POST-OP FOLLOW UP	99024			MMR	90707		NAIL REMOVAL, PARTIAL	11730	
PROLONGED/30-74MIN	99354			PNEUMONIA, >2 Y	90732		NAIL REMOVAL, W/ MATRIX	11750	
SPECIAL REPORTS/FORMS	99080			PNEUMONIA CONJUGATE, <5Y	90669		SKIN TA, 1-15	11200	
DISABILITY/WORKERS COMP	99455			TD, > 7Y	90718		**DENTAL (For practice purposes only)**		
SPECIMIN HANDLING	99000			VARICELLA	90716		PERIODIC ORAL EVALUATION	DE0100	
OFFICE PROCEDURES				**LABORATORY**			COMPREHENSIVE EVALUATION	DE0150	
ANOSCOPY	46600			VENIPUNCTURE	36415		INTRAORAL, PERIAPICAL – 1ST FILM	DE0200	
AUDIOMETRY	92551			BLOOD GLUCOSE, MONITORING DEVICE	82962		INTRAORAL, PERIAPICAL–EACH ADD'L FILM	DE0250	
CERUMEN REMOVAL	69210			BLOOD GLUCOSE, VISUAL DIPSTICK	82948		BITEWING	DE026-	
COLPOSCOPY	54752			CBC, W/ AUTO DIFFERENTIAL	85025		PROPHYLAXIS - ADULT	DE1000	
COLPOSCOPY W/ BIOPSY	57455			CBC, W/O AUTO DIFFRENTIAL	85027		PROPHYLAXIS - CHILD	DE2000	
ECG W/ INTERPRETATION	93000			CHOLESTEROL	82465		PERIODONTAL MAINT.	DE5000	
ECG, RHYTHM STRIP	93040			HEMOOCULT, GUAIAC	82272		RESTORATIVE (ANTERIOR)	DE250-	
ENDOMETRIAL BIOPSY	58100			HEMOCCULT, IMMUNOASSAY	82274		RESTORATIVE (POSTERIOR)	DE260-	
FLEXIBLE SIGMOIDOSCOPY	45330			HEMOGLOBIN A1C	83036		FUSE CROWN-PORC	DE2700	
FLEXIBLE SIGMOIDOSCOPY W/ BIOPSY	45331			LIPID PANEL	80061		RE-CEMENT CROWN	DE2900	
FRACTURE CARE, CAST/SPLINT	29---			LIVER PANEL	80076		CORE BUILD UP INC. PINS	DE3000	
NEBULIZER	94640			KHO PREP (SKIN, HAIR, NAILS)	87220		CORE BUILD UP, PREFAB POST	DE3250	
NEBULIZER DEMO	94664			METABOLIC PANEL, BASIC	80048		LABIAL VENEER	DE3500	
SPIROMETRY	94010			METABOLIC PANEL, COMPHREHENSIVE	80053		CROWN - PORCELAIN FUSED TO GOLD	DE6000	
SPIROMETRY, PRE AND POST	94060			MONONUCLEOSIS	86663		CROWN LENGTHENING	DE4000	
TYMPANOMETRY	92567			PREGNANCY, BLOOD	84702		SURGICAL EXTRACTION	DE7000	
VASECTOMY	55250			PREGNANCY, URINE	81025		IMPACTED EXTRACTION	DE7250	
MEDICATIONS				RENAL PANEL	80069		LTD. ORTHO TREATMENT, ADULT	DE8000	
AMPICILIN, UP TO 500MG	J0290			SEDIMENTATION RATE	85652		ANALGESIA, NITROUS OXIDE	DE9000	

TODAY'S FEE		75.00
AMOUNT RECEIVED		25.00
BALANCE		50.00

 Now complete the review questions for this unit on your Evolve site.

Unit 4 | Payment Posting

A ledger consists of a summary of all payments, charges, and adjustments to a specific patient's account. Sometimes this information needs to be entered manually (e.g., insurance reimbursements or patient payments), but, in the case of entering charges, this information is populated into the patient ledger once the claim has been submitted.

The information in the patient ledger is incredibly important. It not only tracks all credits and debits to a patient account, but also is used to run reports (see Unit 5) and determine when overdue accounts should be sent to collections due to nonpayment. Not keeping records current and not staying on top of outstanding balances is a surefire way to guarantee a practice loses money. So it is not only critical to input data into patient ledgers in a timely manner, but also to review these balances with regularity.

In SimChart for the Medical Office the patient ledger can be accessed through the Info Panel in the Coding & Billing module (Figure 4-1). After selecting the Ledger option from the Info Panel, perform a patient search to open the ledger specific to that account. Within each patient's ledger you'll see information on the transaction date (date the charges or payments were billed/received), the date of service, the provider's name, the service (which could either be a CPT code or practice-defined code to represent a payment), charges, payment, adjustment (if any portion of the charges were written off or adjusted), and the running balance.

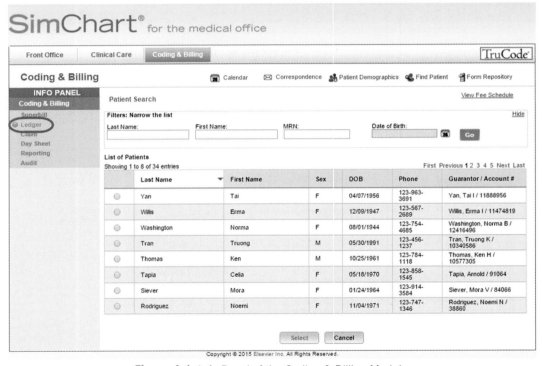

Figure 4-1 Info Panel of the Coding & Billing Module.

Posting Patient Payments

Truong Tran (DOB 05/30/1991) stopped by the medical office to have Jean Burke complete a portion of an application for life insurance. The medical assistant informs Truong Tran that there is a $15.00 fee for this service, and Truong Tran pays the fee with a check (#5671). Document this payment in Truong Tran's ledger.

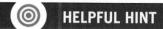 **HELPFUL HINT**

Functions like having paperwork completed or medical records copied typically are not covered by health insurance, and therefore the patient pays the full amount at the time of the service. In cases like these, or other patient payments that might not be tied to a specific date of service, Walden-Martin Family Medical Clinic uses the code "PTPYMTCK" to represent a patient payment on the account made with a check, "PTPYMTCC" to represent a patient payment on the account made with a credit card, and "PTPYMTCSH" to represent a patient payment on the account made with cash.

Measurable Steps

1. Within the Coding & Billing tab, select Ledger from the left Info Panel (Figure 4-2).

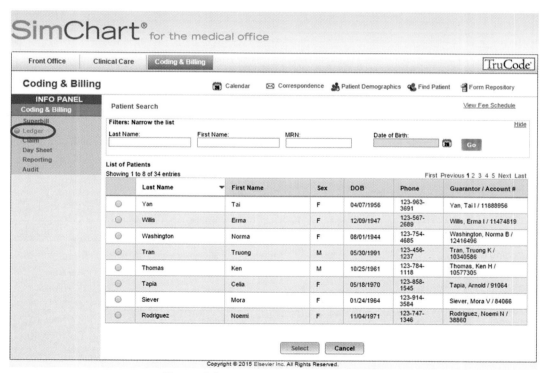

Figure 4-2 Ledger from the left Info Panel.

2. Search for Truong Tran using the Patient Search fields.
3. Select the radio button for Truong Tran and click the Select button.
4. Confirm the autopopulated details in the header.
5. Document the current date in the Transaction Date column using the calendar picker.
6. Document the current date in the DOS column.
7. Select Jean Burke in the Provider dropdown menu.
8. Select the TruCode encoder icon next to the Service column.

9. Enter "insurance form" in the Search field, select CPT Tabular from the dropdown menu, and click the Search button.
10. Click on the 99080 code to expand this code and confirm that it is the most specific code available (Figure 4-3).

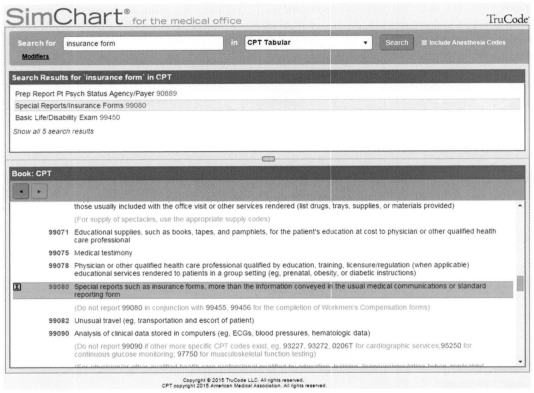

Figure 4-3 Expanding the procedure code.

11. Click the 99080 code for "report preparation" that appears in the tree. This code will autopopulate in the ledger (Figure 4-4).

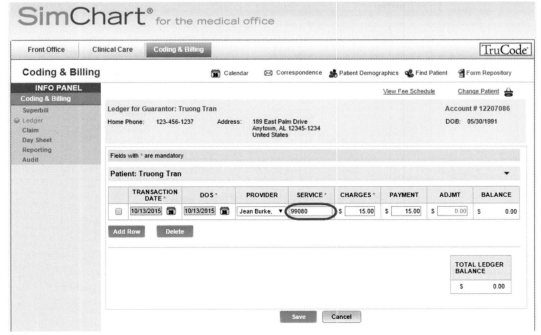

Figure 4-4 Auto-populating the code in the ledger.

Payment Posting

12. Document "15.00" in the Charges column.
13. Document "15.00" in the Payment column.
14. Document "0.00" in the Adjustment column. The balance will autopopulate in the Balance column.
15. Click the Save button.

Payment Posting

Activity

Two additional patients came into the office to have paperwork completed by providers. Please enter their payments in the appropriate patient ledgers.

Patient Name	DOB	Provider	Charges	Payment	Service Code
Maude Crawford	12/22/1946	Martin	$15.00	$15.00	99080
Kyle Reeves	01/01/1996	Walden	$15.00	$15.00	99080

Additionally, three other patients were seen in the office today and made payments. Please enter their payments in the appropriate patient ledgers using the accepted Service Code of PT-PYMTCC to represent patient payments made with a credit card, PTPYMTCK to represent payments made with a check, and PTPYMTCSH to represent payments made with cash.

 HELPFUL HINT

Remember that the charges for office visits will be populated when the superbills are completed, so you will not be documenting them at this time.

Patient Name	DOB	Provider	Charges	Payment	Payment Method
Quinton Brown	02/24/1978	Martin	$0.00	$25.00	Credit Card
Isabella Burgel	07/23/2010	Perez	$0.00	$35.00	Check
Pedro Gomez	07/01/2007	Kahn	$0.00	$35.00	Check

Posting Insurance Reimbursements

Walden-Martin Family Medical Clinic has received an Explanation of Benefits (EOB) from Blue Cross Blue Shield (Figure 4-5). Charles Johnson (DOB 3/3/1958) was seen by Dr. Martin on November 20, 2015. After his copayment and adjustment (the managed care contract agreement discount), Blue Cross Blue Shield reimbursed $33.00 toward Mr. Johnson's account. Monique Jones (DOB 6/23/1985) was another patient seen in the office for a problem-focused office visit and had her knee aspirated. Her two procedures totaled $121.00. After her copayment and adjustment, the reimbursement was $85.00. Post the insurance reimbursements to the individual patient ledgers for these two patients using INSPYMT as the service code.

 HELPFUL HINT

Insurance companies might provide a single EOB with multiple patients listed as seen in Figure 4-5, or an insurance carrier might provide individual EOBs with just one patient listed on each (see the first EOB after this assignment). Pay close attention to the documents to ensure you don't miss any payments!

BLUE CROSS BLUE SHIELD
1234 Insurance Place
Anytown, AL 12345-1234

Provider: James Martin
Check #: 641358
Check Date: 12/15/2015
Check Amount: $118.00

Walden-Martin
1234 Anystreet
Anytown, AL 13245-1234

DOS	Procedure	Billed	Contract Adjustment	Co-Pay	Deductible	Paid
NAME: Charles Johnson				**ID#: 46859J**		
11/20/2015	99214	$65.00	$7.00	$25.00	$0.00	$33.00
	CLAIM TOTALS:	$65.00	$7.00	$25.00	$0.00	$33.00
NAME: Monique Jones				**ID#: MJ4468871**		
11/16/2015	99212	$32.00	$4.00	$25.00	$0.00	$3.00
11/16/2015	20610	$89.00	$7.00	$0.00	$0.00	$82.00
	CLAIM TOTALS:	$121.00	$11.00	$25.00	$0.00	$85.00

Figure 4-5 Blue Cross Blue Shield Explanation of Benefits (EOB).

Measurable Steps

1. Within the Coding & Billing tab, select Ledger from the left Info Panel.
2. Search for Charles Johnson using the Patient Search fields.
3. Select the radio button for Charles Johnson and click the Select button.

4. Confirm the autopopulated details in the header (Figure 4-6).

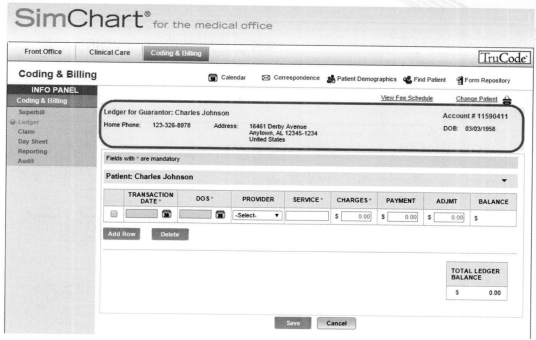

Figure 4-6 Confirm Charles Johnson's details in the header.

5. Document the current date in the Transaction Date column using the calendar picker.
6. Document the Date of Service from the EOB in the DOS column.
7. Select "James Martin" from the Provider dropdown menu.
8. Document "INSPYMT" in the Service column.
9. Document "0.00" in the Charges column.

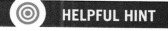

HELPFUL HINT

Remember that the service charges and copayment were already logged at the time of the patient's visit, so it is important to not duplicate this entry. The Explanation of Benefits only provides information on what the insurance carrier paid, so that is the only payment that should be logged at this time.

10. Document "33.00" from the Claim Totals line on the EOB into the Payment column.
11. Document "-7.00" from the Claim Totals line in the Adjustment column. The balance will auto-populate in the Balance column.

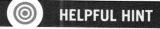

HELPFUL HINT

Remember to use a "-" with the adjustment to ensure that it subtracts from the total balance!

12. Click the Save button.
13. Search for Monique Jones using the Patient Search fields.
14. Select the radio button for Monique Jones and click the Select button.

Payment Posting

15. Confirm the autopopulated details in the header (Figure 4-7).

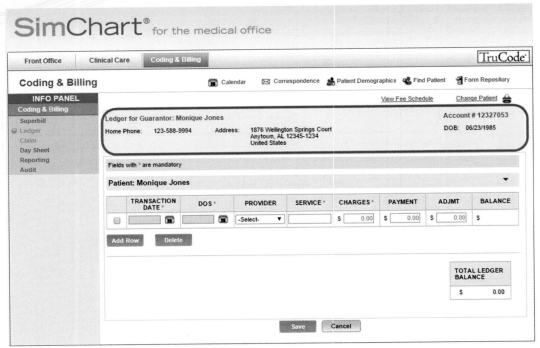

Figure 4-7 Confirm Monique Jones' details in the header.

16. Document the current date in the Transaction Date column using the calendar picker.
17. Document the Date of Service from the EOB in the DOS column.
18. Select "James Martin" from the Provider dropdown menu.
19. Document "INSPYMT" in the Service column.
20. Document "0.00" in the Charges column.
21. Document "85.00" from the Claim Totals line on the EOB into the Payment column.

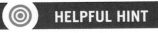 **HELPFUL HINT**

Because the purpose is documenting the total payment from the insurance company, rather than the specific procedure codes that were already documented on the date of the visit, you don't have to submit separate lines for different procedures when posting insurance reimbursements. Instead use the totals for the entire grouping of procedures for a patient on the specific date of service.

22. Document "-11.00" from the Claim Totals line in the Adjustment column. The balance will autopopulate in the Balance column.
23. Click the Save button.

Payment Posting

Activity

Use the following EOBs to post insurance payments to the appropriate patients' ledgers.

MEDICARE

1234 Insurance Road
Anytown, AL 12345-1234

Walden-Martin
1234 Anystreet
Anytown, AL 13245-1234

Provider: James Martin
Check #: 452189
Check Date: 12/28/15
Check Amount: $70.00

DOS	Procedure	Billed	Contract Adjustment	Co-Pay	Deductible	Paid
NAME: Maude Crawford				**ID#: 479376613A**		
12/4/15	99397	$120.00	$50.00	$0.00	$0.00	$70.00
	CLAIM TOTALS:	$120.00	$50.00	$0.00	$0.00	$70.00

MetLife

1234 Insurance Avenue
Anytown, AL 12345-1234

Walden-Martin
1234 Anystreet
Anytown, AL 13245-1234

Provider:	Talibah Nasser
Patient DOB:	07/09/1980
Provider:	Jean Burke
Paid Date:	12/04/15
Check Number:	N/A

DOS	Procedure	Billed	Contract Adjustment	Co-Pay	Deductible	Paid
11/9/15	Q0091	$52.00	$18.00	$25.00	$9.00	$0.00
	TOTALS:	$52.00	$18.00	$25.00	$9.00	$0.00

BLUE CROSS
BLUE SHIELD
1234 Insurance Place
Anytown, AL 12345-1234

Provider: James Martin
Check #: 369856
Check Date: 11/23/15
Check Amount: $68.00

Walden-Martin
1234 Anystreet
Anytown, AL 13245-1234

DOS	Procedure	Billed	Contract Adjustment	Co-Pay	Deductible	Paid
NAME: Julia Berkley				**ID#: JB7114521**		
10/28/15	99212	$32.00	$7.00	$25.00	$0.00	$0.00
	CLAIM TOTALS:	$32.00	$7.00	$25.00	$0.00	$0.00
NAME: Malcolm Little				**ID#: 46859J**		
10/22/15	99205	$119.00	$26.00	$25.00	$0.00	$68.00
	CLAIM TOTALS:	$119.00	$26.00	$25.00	$0.00	$68.00

NOTE: To complete the remaining activities, you'll need to make sure that you've added the following patients from Unit 2 to the system: Jessie Baer, Boyd Dubois, Kim Nguyen, and Lou Thao.

AETNA DENTAL PPO

Provider: Patrick Taylor
Check #: 245769
Check Date: 12/18/2015
Check Amount: $1205.25

1234 Insurance Way
Anytown, AL 12345-1234

Walden-Martin
1234 Anystreet
Anytown, AL 13245-1234

DOS	Procedure	Billed	Contract Adjustment	Co-Insurance	Deductible	Paid
NAME: Ahmad Reuven				**ID#: RH6659862**		
11/11/15	DE3500	$847.00	$150.00	$174.25	$0.00	$522.75
11/11/15	DE2700	$975.00	$195.00	$195.00	$0.00	$585.00
	CLAIM TOTALS:	$1,822.00	$345.00	$369.25	$0.00	$1107.75
NAME: Lou Thao				**ID#: 46859J**		
11/13/15	DE0100	$36.00	$12.00	$6.00	$0.00	$18.00
11/13/15	DE1000	$64.00	$17.00	$11.75	$0.00	$35.25
	CLAIM TOTALS:	$100.00	$29.00	$17.75	$0.00	$53.25

Total Medical Insurance

1255 Insurance Avenue
Anytown, AL 12345-1234

Walden-Martin
1234 Anystreet
Anytown, AL 13245-1234

Provider: Boyd Dubois
Patient DOB: 04/30/1958
Provider: David Kahn
Paid Date: 12/22/15
Check Number: 165894

DOS	Procedure	Billed	Contract Adjustment	Co-Pay	Deductible	Paid
12/01/15	11200	$49.00	$9.00	$25.00	$0.00	$15.00
	TOTALS:	$49.00	$9.00	$25.00	$0.00	$15.00

Helping Hand

1255 Insurance Way
Anytown, AL 12345-1234

Walden-Martin
1234 Anystreet
Anytown, AL 13245-1234

Provider: Jessie Baer
Patient DOB: 05/25/1995
Provider: Angela Perez
Paid Date: 11/30/15
Check Number: 845796

DOS	Procedure	Billed	Contract Adjustment	Co-Insurance	Deductible	Paid
11/02/15	99202	$50.00	$12.50	$9.38	$0.00	$28.12
11/02/15	85027	$25.00	$6.25	$4.69	$0.00	$14.06
11/02/15	36415	$10.00	$2.50	$1.87	$0.00	$5.63
	TOTALS:	$85.00	$21.25	$15.94	$0.00	$47.81

Delta Dental

1255 Insurance Boulevard
Anytown, AL 12345-1234

Walden-Martin
1234 Anystreet
Anytown, AL 13245-1234

Provider: Kim Ngyuen
Patient DOB: 10/01/1954
Provider: Patrick Taylor
Paid Date: 12/10/15
Check Number: 54896

DOS	Procedure	Billed	Contract Adjustment	Co-Insurance	Deductible	Paid
11/6/15	DE3500	$847.00	$211.75	$158.81	$0.00	$476.44
11/6/15	DE2700	$975.00	$243.75	$182.81	$0.00	$548.44
11/6/15	DE2700	$975.00	$243.75	$182.81	$0.00	$548.44
11/6/15	DE2700	$975.00	$243.75	$182.81	$0.00	$548.44
	TOTALS:	$3,772.00	$943.00	$707.24	$0.00	$2,121.76

 Now complete the Review Questions for this unit on your Evolve site.

Unit 5 | Reports

Ledgers are specific to patients, whereas the **Day Sheet** is a listing of all charges billed and payments received by the practice on a particular day. In this way payments received from multiple patients on a given day will all be logged on the same day sheet, which is then used to complete bank deposit slips at the end of the day and for reporting and practice analysis in the short and long term. Using this data to create monthly, quarterly, and annual reports can give a larger picture of how the practice is running.

In SimChart for the Medical Office the day sheet can be accessed through the Info Panel in the Coding & Billing module (Figure 5-1). After Day Sheet is selected from the Info Panel, a new sheet will open, but previously saved day sheets can be accessed by clicking on the Saved Day Sheets tab at the top of the screen.

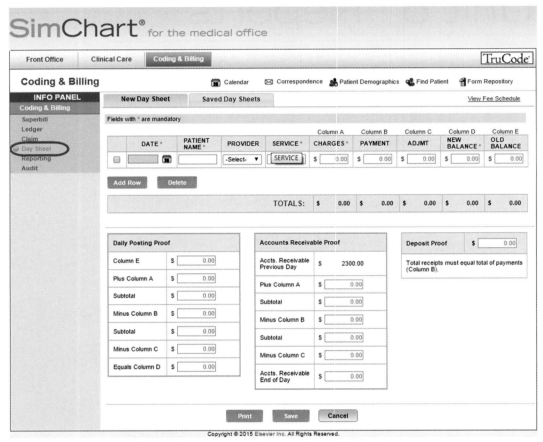

Figure 5-1 Info Panel of the Coding & Billing Module.

In addition to broadening the view from specific patients and encounters with the day sheet, a practice manager can run a number of reports to assist with the accounting of a practice. An **activity report** summarizes the patient activity in an office by either procedure or diagnosis. This report could assist in determining the most common procedures used in a medical office in order to plan the space accordingly. For example, if a significant number of patients are seen for sigmoidoscopies, but there is only one exam room that has the proper equipment for this type of exam, this report could be used to justify reallocation of office space and purchase of additional equipment. Another example of the usefulness of activity reports is if new information on osteoporosis is published and one of the providers wants to send a letter to relevant patients, a report could be run on diagnosis codes related to osteoporosis to target the correct audience.

Aging reports are one of the most useful tools of a medical office. These reports can be broken down by patient or insurance company and will provide a summary of all outstanding balances within a certain period. These balances are further broken down by how far past due they are. The most important aspect of keeping a business running is to ensure that payments are made in a timely manner, and an aging report is the best way to make sure that payments are not delayed and to determine when it is appropriate to send accounts to collections. A practice should run these reports regularly to follow up with outstanding debts from both patients and insurance carriers.

In SimChart for the Medical Office the reporting functionality can be accessed through the Info Panel in the Coding & Billing module (Figure 5-2). After selecting Reporting from the Info Panel, you can select the type of report you would like using the dropdown menu.

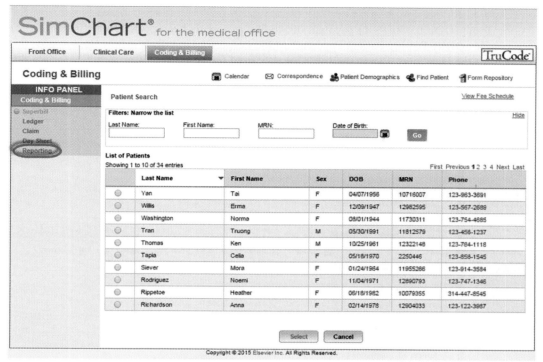

Figure 5-2 Reporting in the Left Info Panel.

Posting Patient Payments to the Day Sheet

Truong Tran's (DOB 05/30/1991) payment of $15.00 has already been posted to his patient ledger (see sample activity Posting Patient Payments to the Ledger in Unit 4). It is now time to post this payment to the Day Sheet. Please use the same date used on Truong's ledger to indicate when this payment was received in the practice. Truong does not have a previous balance on his account.

Measurable Steps

1. Select Day Sheet from the left Info Panel (Figure 5-3).

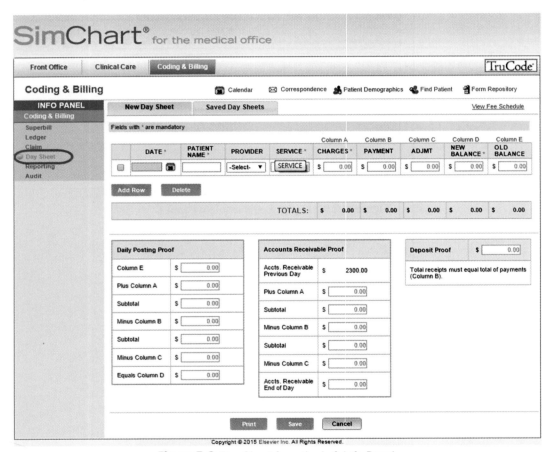

Figure 5-3 Day Sheet from the Left Info Panel.

2. Document the date of Truong's payment in the Date column using the calendar picker.
3. Document "Truong Tran" in the Patient column.
4. Select "Jean Burke" in the Provider dropdown menu.
5. Document "99080" in the Service column.
6. Document "15.00" in the Charges column.
7. Document "15.00" in the Payment column.
8. Leave the Adjustment column blank.
9. Because Truong paid the entirety of the $15.00 charges and does not have an old balance, document $0.00 in the Old Balance column and the New Balance column.
10. Click the Save button (Figure 5-4).

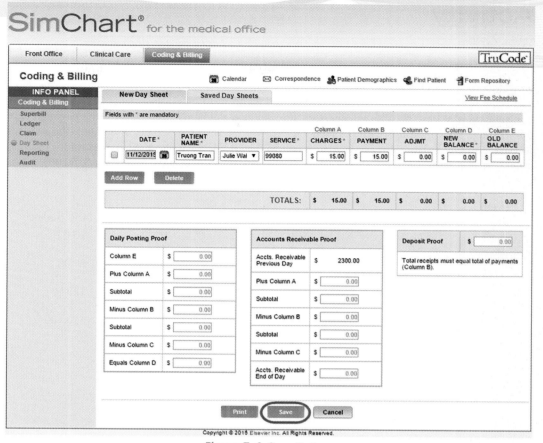

Figure 5-4 Save Button.

Activity

Now document the charges and payments below on the same day sheet you began with Truong. Note that because these are patient payments, there will be no insurance adjustments (ADJMT column). For patients who have no Old Balance, the New Balance will be the charges with the payment subtracted (e.g., for Quinton Brown the New Balance will be $80.00 − $25.00, or $55.00). For patients who have an Old Balance, the New Balance will be the Old Balance plus the Charges minus the Payment (e.g., for Pedro Gomez the New Balance will be $100.00 + $75.00 − $25.00, or $150.00).

Patient Name	DOB	Provider	Charges	Payment	Service Code	Old Balance
Quinton Brown	02/24/1978	Taylor	$80.00	$25.00	99395	$0.00
Maude Crawford	12/22/1946	Martin	$15.00	$15.00	99080	$0.00
Isabella Burgel	07/23/2010	Perez	$75.00	$25.00	99392	$25.00
Pedro Gomez	07/01/2007	Kahn	$75.00	$25.00	99392	$100.00
Kyle Reeves	01/01/1996	Walden	$15.00	$15.00	99080	$0.00

Posting Insurance Payments to the Day Sheet

On the same day that the charges and payments for the previous activities were logged Walden-Martin Family Medical Clinic received an explanation of benefits (EOB) and check from MetLife (Figure 5-5) for an office visit from Anna Richardson (DOB 02/14/1978). Anna neglected to make her copayment of $25.00 at the time of her visit, so prior to this payment her Old Balance is $43.00. Please log this payment on the correct Day Sheet.

MetLife

1234 Insurance Avenue
Anytown, AL 12345-1234

Walden-Martin
1234 Anystreet
Anytown, AL 13245-1234

Provider: Anna Richardson
Patient DOB: 02/14/1978
Provider: James Martin
Paid Date: 12/01/2015
Check Number: 341183

DOS	Procedure	Billed	Contract Adjustment	Co-Pay	Deductible	Paid
10/28/2015	99213	$43.00	$8.00	$25.00	$0.00	$10.00

Figure 5-5 MetLife Explanation of Benefits (EOB).

Measurable Steps

1. Select Day Sheet from the left Info Panel.
2. Click on the Saved Day Sheets tab and use the dropdown menu to find the day sheet used in the previous activity.
3. Use the calendar picker to select the same date as the previous activity in the Date column.
4. Select the Add Row button and document "Anna Richardson" in the Patient Name column.
5. Select James Martin from the provider dropdown menu.
6. Document the INSPYMT in the Service column.

 HELPFUL HINT

INSPYMT is the code Walden-Martin Family Medical Clinic uses to designate insurance payments. The CPT code from the Service column of the EOB is not used because this code was already documented during the patient's date of service.

7. Document "0.00" in the Charges column.
8. Document "10.00" in the Payment column.
9. Document "8.00" from the Contract Adjustment column on the EOB in the ADJMT column.
10. Document Anna's previous balance of 43.00 in the Old Balance. The New Balance should be 25.00.
11. Click the Save button (Figure 5-6).

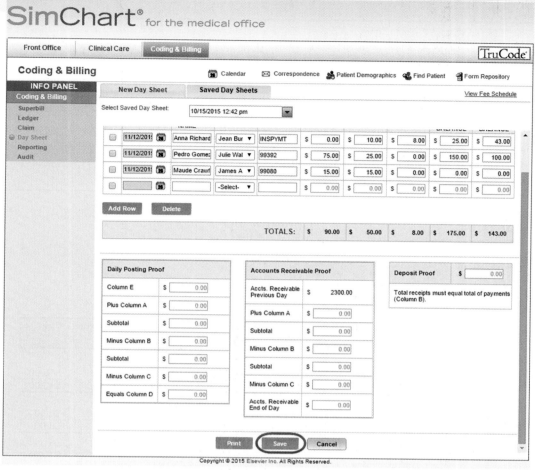

Figure 5-6 Save Button.

◎ HELPFUL HINT

Selecting the Print button will open the Day Sheet into a new tab where you will also have the opportunity to right-click and save the file into your records. This is a useful tool if your instructor asks for you to submit your work in either print or electronic format.

Activity

A number of the doctors were out of the office for consultations or surgeries on December 1, 2015, so it was determined the office would be closed to patients to catch up on administrative work. However, Walden-Martin Family Medical Clinic received the following EOB and check from Aetna. Please document these payments in a new day sheet for this date. (NOTE: None of these patients have previous balances, but because of deductibles, some may end up with a New Balance.) Save your work and print a copy if your instructor requires it.

AETNA

1234 Insurance Way
Anytown, AL 12345-1234

Walden-Martin
1234 Anystreet
Anytown, AL 13245-1234

Provider: James Martin
Check #: 264168
Check Date: 12/01/2015
Check Amount: $50.00

DOS	Procedure	Billed	Contract Adjustment	Co-Pay	Deductible	Paid
NAME: Ella Rainwater				**ID#: CB3247462**		
11/02/2015	G0101	$79.00	$14.00	$25.00	$0.00	$40.00
	CLAIM TOTALS:	$79.00	$14.00	$25.00	$0.00	$40.00
NAME: Noemi Rodriguez				**ID#: NR5006789**		
11/06/2015	99213	$43.00	$8.00	$25.00	$10.00	$0.00
	CLAIM TOTALS:	$43.00	$8.00	$25.00	$10.00	$0.00
NAME: Al Neviaser				**ID#: AN4235543**		
10/26/2015	99213	$43.00	$8.00	$25.00	$0.00	$10.00
	CLAIM TOTALS:	$43.00	$8.00	$25.00	$0.00	$10.00

Generating a Bank Deposit Slip

You were out of the office yesterday and were unable to make the daily deposit to the bank at the end of the day. Walden-Martin Family Medical Clinic saw a number of patients yesterday, some of whom have paid copayments, fees, or account balances. Additionally, you've received a couple of reimbursement checks from insurance carriers. The cash and checks received were all stored in the safe for you to deposit first thing in the morning. Assuming that all of these payments have been logged in the patient ledgers and on the day sheet, complete the bank deposit slip using the following payment information:

- Amma Patel (DOB 01/14/1988) paid $25.00 by check
- Celia Tapia (DOB 05/18/1970) paid $25.00 cash
- Charles Johnson (DOB 03/03/1958) paid $50.00 by check
- Diego Lupez (DOB 08/01/1982) paid $25.00 by check
- Ella Rainwater (DOB 07/11/1959) paid $25.00 by check
- Janine Butler (DOB 04/25/1968) paid $15.00 by check
- Quinton Brown (DOB 02/24/1978) paid $43.00 cash
- Tai Yan (DOB 04/07/1956) paid $15.00 cash
- Talibah Nasser (DOB 07/09/1980) paid $25.00 by check
- Truong Tran (DOB 05/30/1991) paid $25.00 by check
- Anna Richardson (DOB 02/14/1978) paid $15.00 cash
- Aetna (insurance reimbursement) paid $256.00 by check
- Medicare (insurance reimbursement) paid $372.00 by check

Measurable Steps

1. Click the Form Repository icon and select Bank Deposit Slip from the Office Forms section (Figure 5-7).

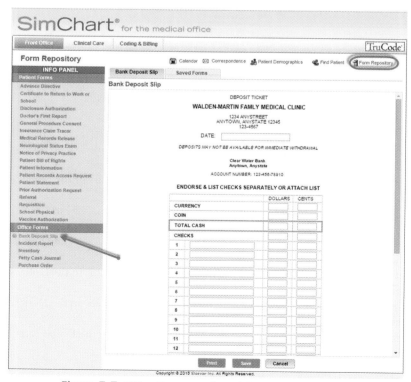

Figure 5-7 Office Forms section of the Form Repository.

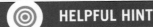

HELPFUL HINT

Although the payments were all received yesterday, you will be putting today's date on the bank deposit slip because the date should reflect the day the deposit is made.

2. Document today's date in the Date field.
3. Add up all of the cash payments and document this total into the Currency row.
4. Enter the total you came up with in step 3 into the Total Cash row.
5. In the first row beneath the Checks heading, document "Amma Patel" in the first column, "25" in the Dollars column, and "00" in the Cents column (Figure 5-8).

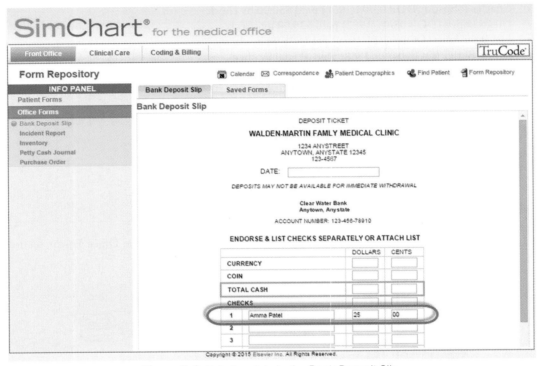

Figure 5-8 Entering data in the Bank Deposit Slip.

6. In the second row, document "Charles Johnson" in the first column, "50" in the Dollars column, and "00" in the Cents column.
7. In the third row, document "Diego Lupez" in the first column, "25" in the Dollars column, and "00" in the Cents column.
8. In the fourth row, document "Ella Rainwater" in the first column, "25" in the Dollars column, and "00" in the Cents column.
9. In the fifth row, document "Janine Butler" in the first column, "15" in the Dollars column, and "00" in the Cents column.
10. In the sixth row, document "Talibah Nasser" in the first column, "25" in the Dollars column, and "00" in the Cents column.
11. In the seventh row, document "Truong Tran" in the first column, "25" in the Dollars column, and "00" in the Cents column.
12. In the eighth row, document "Aetna" in the first column, "256" in the Dollars column, and "00" in the Cents column.

13. In the ninth row, document "Medicare" in the first column, "372" in the Dollars column, and "00" in the Cents column.
14. Add up all of the checks you've logged and enter this total into the Checks column near the top of the slip.
15. Add the amount from the Total Cash row with the amount from the Checks row and document that number in the Total From Attached List field.
16. Document "10" in the Total Items field.
17. Click the Save button.

Activity

At the end of the day today, the following payments were received from patients and insurance providers. Please create the bank deposit slip for the nightly deposit. Make sure to save your work.

 HELPFUL HINT

After completing this activity you will have two bank deposit slips with the same date. Note that SimChart for the Medical Office time stamps your slips when they are saved so you will be able to tell which deposit was the morning deposit (of the previous day's payments) and which was the evening deposit (of the current day's payments).

- Al Neviaser (DOB 06/21/1968) paid $15.00 cash
- Julia Berkley (DOB 07/05/1992) paid $85.00 by check
- Walter Biller (DOB 01/04/1970) paid $15.00 by check
- Robert Caudill (DOB 10/31/1940) paid $18.00 by check
- Jesus Garcia (DOB 09/09/1988) paid $25.00 by check
- Maddy Martin (DOB 03/12/1983) paid $25.00 cash
- Boyd Dubois (DOB 04/30/1958) paid $15.00 cash
- Kim Nguyen (DOB 10/01/1954) paid $27.00 by check
- Health First (insurance reimbursement) paid $68.00 by check
- Total Medical Insurance (insurance reimbursement) paid $123.00 by check

Running an Activity Report

All of the doctors in the practice are interested in getting feedback from patients new to the office between August 1, 2015 and July 31, 2016. They have asked you to run an activity report for all new outpatient office visits for that 12-month period. Use the reporting feature in SimChart for the Medical Office to generate this information for the doctors.

Measurable Steps

1. Click on the Coding & Billing tab at the top of the screen.
2. Select Reporting from the left Info Panel.
3. Select Procedure Usage from the Report dropdown menu (Figure 5-9).

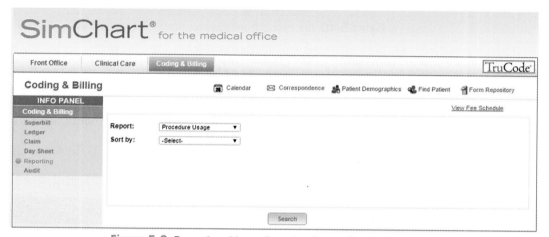

Figure 5-9 Procedure Usage from the Report Dropdown Menu.

4. Select Patient from the Sort By dropdown menu.
5. Select the radio button next to All Active Patients.
6. Place the cursor in the first row under Procedure Code(s) to activate the TruCode encoder (Figure 5-10).

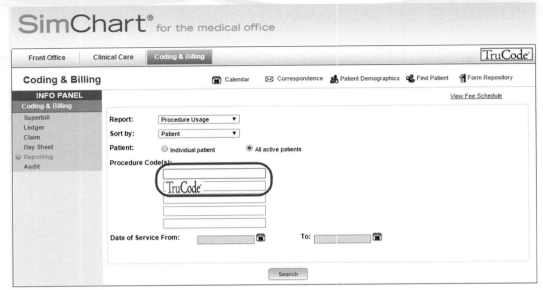

Figure 5-10 Accessing TrueCode encoder.

7. Type "office visit new" in the search field and select CPT Tabular from the dropdown menu and click Search.
8. Select the Show all 25 search results hyperlink to show all new office visits in the menu. Note that there are five diagnosis codes for new outpatient office visits. Select the first, 99201.
9. Select the 99201 hyperlink in the bottom pane to ensure it is the most specific code. It will auto-populate in the first Procedure Code(s) field of your activity report.
10. Use the same process to populate the remaining four new outpatient office visits in the remaining four fields under Procedure Code(s).

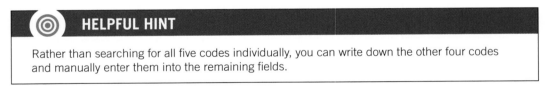

HELPFUL HINT

Rather than searching for all five codes individually, you can write down the other four codes and manually enter them into the remaining fields.

11. Use the calendar picker to select August 1, 2015 in the Date of Service From field.
12. Use the calendar picker to select July 31, 2016 in the To field.
13. Click Search. The report will generate as a portable document format (PDF) file in your browser.
14. Save the PDF for your records. Your instructor may ask you to submit your work electronically or print out a copy.

Activity

The doctors were so pleased with your results on the office visit report that they would like to do the same with new patient wellness visits for the same time period (August 1, 2015 through July 31, 2016). Please run an activity report for all new patients that were seen for "preventative medicine new." Note that there are more than five procedure codes so you will have to run two reports to cover all of the applicable codes. Save these reports to your files or print them.

Running an Aging Report

Walden-Martin Family Medical Clinic has hired an intern for the billing department. He is going to assist in clearing up outstanding balances with the different insurance providers. In order to get the intern started, you need to run an aging report on Blue Cross/Blue Shield.

Measurable Steps

1. Click on the Coding & Billing tab at the top of the screen.
2. Select Reporting from the left Info Panel.
3. Select Aging from the Report dropdown menu (Figure 5-11).

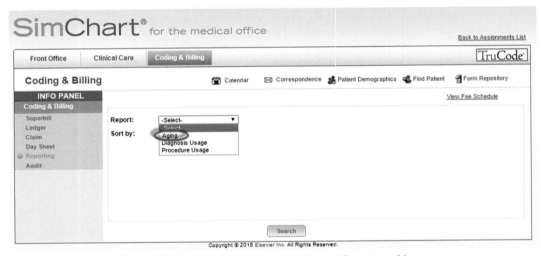

Figure 5-11 Aging Report from the Report Dropdown Menu.

4. Select Insurance from the Sort By dropdown menu.
5. Select Blue Cross/Blue Shield from the Insurance dropdown menu.
6. Use the calendar picker to select August 1, 2015 in the Date of Service From field.
7. Use the calendar picker to select July 31, 2016 in the To field.
8. Click Search. The report will generate as a portable document format (PDF) file in your browser.
9. Save the PDF for your records. Your instructor may ask you to submit your work electronically or print out a copy.

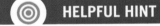 **HELPFUL HINT**

The reports that you run in SimChart for the Medical Office are not saved or stored anywhere within the application. It is a good idea to right click on your report and select "Save as" to keep a copy in your files to submit electronically or print and hand in to your instructor.

Activity

The intern did such a good job clearing up Blue Cross/Blue Shield balances that you've decided to have him follow up on any outstanding balances with Medicare. Run an aging report for Medicare balances for the same time period. Save this report to your files or print it.

 Now complete the Review Questions for this unit on your Evolve site.

Unit 6 | Comprehensive Cases

Now you will experience the entire process of a patient visit from registration and scheduling appointments through the billing and reporting process.

Case #1

Marcie Anderson calls first thing this morning needing a 6-month cleaning as soon as possible because she is leaving the country next week for an extended trip. You look at the schedule and see that Dr. Taylor has an opening at 10:30 this morning because of a cancelled appointment. Using Marcie's patient information form (Figure 6-1), enter her information into the system and schedule her for 45 minutes with Dr. Taylor and his hygienist beginning at 10:30.

WALDEN-MARTIN
FAMILY MEDICAL CLINIC
1234 ANYSTREET | ANYTOWN, ANYSTATE 12345
PHONE 123-123-1234 | FAX 123-123-5678

JULIE WALDEN MD
JAMES MARTIN MD
DAVID KAHN MD
ANGELA PEREZ MD
PATRICK TAYLOR DDS
JEAN BURKE NP

DENTAL

PATIENT INFORMATION

First Name	MI	Last Name	Date of Birth	Sex
Marcie		Anderson	5/8/83	F

SSN	Home Phone	Work Phone	Cell
651-58-1705	123-865-0987		

Home Address	City	State	Zip
901 Boxcart Dr	Anytown	AL	12345-1234

Marital Status	Employer	Driver's License #
Single	Anytown Advertising Agency	SH36693862

Emergency Contact	Relationship to Patient	Phone Number
Diane Anderson		123-865-5555

RESPONSIBLE PARTY INFORMATION   SELF ☑

First Name	MI	Last Name	Date of Birth	Sex
Marcie		Anderson	5/8/83	F

SSN	Home Phone	Work Phone	Cell
651-58-1705	123-865-0987		

Home Address	City	State	Zip
901 Boxcart Dr	Anytown	AL	12345-1234

Employer	Relationship to Patient
Anytown Advertising Agency	Self

DENTAL INSURANCE INFORMATION

Primary Insurance Carrier	Phone Number
Self Pay	

Address	City	State	Zip

Policy Holder Name (if different from patient)	Phone	Date of Birth	Sex

Policy Number	Group Number

I hereby give lifetime authorization for payment of insurance benefits to be made directly to Walden-Martin Medical Group, and any assisting physicians, for services rendered. I understand that I am financially responsible for all charges whether or not they are covered by insurance. In the event of default, I agree to pay all costs of collection, and reasonable attorney's fees. I hereby authorize this healthcare provider to release all information necessary to secure the payment of benefits. I further agree that a photocopy of this agreement shall be as valid as the original.

Signature	Date
Marcie Anderson	

Figure 6-1 Patient Information Form and Insurance Card for Marcie Anderson.

Dr. Taylor's hygienist has asked you to fill in the dental history of the patient using her notes (Box 6-1). Use the instructions below to complete this:

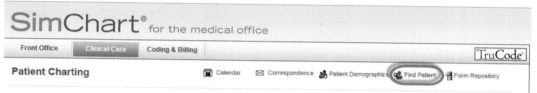

BOX 6-1

Marcie Anderson's Dental History

Last Dental Exam: *01/05/2015*
Name of Dentist: *Mary Rodgers, DDS*
Dental Issue: *none*
Notes: *All four wisdom teeth removed approximately 5 years ago.*

1. Click the Find Patient button at the top of the screen (Figure 6-2).

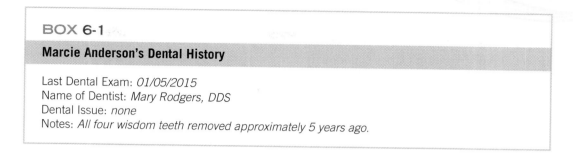

Figure 6-2 Find Patient Icon.

2. Enter Anderson into the Last Name search field and select the Go button.
3. If Marcie Anderson was registered correctly, her name should populate in the search results. Select the radio button next to it and click Select.
4. Select Office Visit from the left Info Panel.
5. Select today's date from the calendar picker.
6. Select 6 Month Visit from the Visit Type dropdown menu.
7. Select Patrick Taylor from the provider dropdown menu and click the Save button.
8. Select Health History from the Record dropdown menu.
9. Select the tab titled Dental History.
10. Select the Add New button.
11. Enter the data from Box 6-1 into the correct fields in the box that pops up.
12. Click the Save Button.

At the end of the day, Marcie's encounter is coded, and you are provided with the following paper encounter form to complete her superbill within SimChart for the Medical Office. Make sure to post her charges to the day sheet.

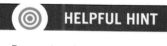
HELPFUL HINT

Remember that claims are not submitted for patients who are self-pay. Therefore you do not have to submit a claim for Marcie Anderson.

WALDEN-MARTIN
FAMILY MEDICAL CLINIC
1234 ANYSTREET | ANYTOWN, ANYSTATE 12345
PHONE 123-123-1234 | FAX 123-123-5678

JULIE WALDEN MD
JAMES MARTIN MD
DAVID KAHN MD
ANGELA PEREZ MD
(PATRICK TAYLOR DDS)
JEAN BURKE NP

Patient Name: Anderson, Marcie
DOS: [TODAY]
Diagnoses 1):
2):
3):
4):

SERVICE	CODE		PRICE	SERVICE	CODE	PRICE	SERVICE	CODE	PRICE
OFFICE VISIT	New	Est.		MEDICATIONS CONT'D			LABORATORY CONT'D		
MINIMAL OFFICE VISIT (OV)	99201	99211		B-12, UP TO 1,000MCG	J3420		STREP, RAPID	87880	
PROBLEM FOCUSED OV	99202	99212		EPINEPHINE, UP TO 1ML	J0170		STREP CULTURE	87081	
EXPANDED OV	99203	99213		KENALOG, 10MG	J3301		TB	87116	
DETAILED OV	99204	99214		LIDCAINE, 10MG	J2001		UA, COMPLETE, NON-AUTOMATED, MICRO	81000	
COMPHREHENSIVE OV	99205	99215		PROGESTERONE, 150MG	J1055		UA, W/O MICRO NON-AUTOMATED	81002	
WELLNESS VISIT	New	Est.		RECEPHIN, 250MG	J0696		UA, W/ MICRO, NON-AUTOMATED	81001	
WELL VISIT < 1 Y	99381	99391		TESTOSTERONE, 200MG	J1080		URINE COLONY COUNT	87086	
WELL VISIT 1-4 Y	99382	99392		TIGAN, UP TO 200MG	J3250		WET MOUNT/KOH	87210	
WELL VISIT 5-11 Y	99383	99393		TORADOL, 15MG	J1885		INPATIENT/OUTPATIENT PROCEDURES		
WELL VISIT 12-17 Y	99384	99394		NORMAL SALINE, 1000CC	J7030		UPPER GI ENDOSCOPY	43235	
WELL VISIT 18-39 Y	99385	99395		PHENERGAN, UP TO 50MG	J2550		UPPER GI ENDOSCOPY W/ BIOPSY	43239	
WELL VISIT 40-64 Y	99386	99396		IMMUNIZATIONS & INJECTIONS			UPPER GI ENDOSCOPY W/ GUIDE WIRE	43248	
WELL VISIT 65 Y+	99387	99397		ALLERGEN, ONE	95115		UPPER GI ENDOSCOPY W/ BALLOON	43249	
PREVENTATIVE SERVICES				ALLERGEN, MULTIPLE	95117		COLONOSCOPY	45378	
PAP	Q0091			IMM ADMIN, ONE	90471		COLONOSCOPY W/ BIOPSY	45380	
PELVIC & BREAST	G0101			IMM ADMIN, EACH ADD'L	90472		COLONOSCOPY W/ BIOPSY REMOVAL	45384	
PROSTATE/PSA	G0103			IMM ADMIN, INTRANASAL, ONE	90473		COLONOSCOPY W/ SNARE REMOVAL	45385	
TOBACCO COUNSELING/3-10MIN	99406			IMM ADMIN, INTRANASAL, EACH ADD'L	90475		SKIN PROCEDURES		
TOBACCO COUNSELING/>10MIN	99407			INJECTION, JOINT, SMALL	206--		BURN CARE, INITIAL	16000	
WELCOME TO MEDICARE EXAM	G0366			INJECTION, THER/PROPH/DIAG	90772		FROEIGN BODY, SKIN, SIMPLE	10120	
ECG W/ WELCOME TO MEDICARE EXAM	G0366			INJECTION, TRIGGER POINT	20552		FOREIGN BODY, SKIN, COMPLEX	12121	
FLEXIBLE SIGMOIDOSCOPY	G0104			VACCINES			I&D, ABSCESS	10060	
HEMOCCULT, GUAIAC	G0107			DT, <7 Y	90702		I&D, HEMATOMA/SEROMA	10140	
FLU ADMINISTRATION	G0008			DTP	90701		LCERATION REPAIR, SIMPLE	120--	
PENUMONIA ADMINISTRATION	G0009			DTAP, <7 Y	90700		LACERATION REPAIR, LAYERED	120--	
CONSULTATION/PRE-OP CLEARANCE				FLU, 6-35 MONTHS	90657		LESION, BIOPSY, ONE	11100	
EXPANDED PROBLEM FOCUSED	99242			FLU, 3Y+	90658		LESION, BIOPSY, EACH ADD'L	11101	
DETAILED	99243			HEP A, PED/ADOL, 2 DOSE	90633		LESION, DEST., BENIGN 1-14	17110	
COMPREHENSIVE/MOD COMPLEXITY	99244			HEP A, ADULT	90632		LESION DEST., PRE-MAL., SINGLE	17000	
COMPREHENSIVE/HIGH COMPLEXITY	99245			HEP B, PED/ADOL, 3 DOSE	90744		LESION DEST., PRE-MAL., EACH ADD'L	17003	
OTHER SERVICES				HEP B, ADULT	90746		LESION, EXCISION BENIGN	114--	
AFTER POSTED HOURS	99050			HEP B-HIB	90748		LESION, EXCISION, MALIGNANT	116--	
EVENING/WEEKEND APPT.	99051			HIB, 4 DOSE	90645		LESION, PARING/CUTTING, ONE	11055	
HOME HEALTH CERTIFICATION	G0180			HPV	90649		LESION PARING/CUTTING 2-4	11056	
HOME HEALTH RECERTIFICATION	G0179			IPV	90713		LESION, SHAVE	113--	
POST-OP FOLLOW UP	99024			MMR	90707		NAIL REMOVAL, PARTIAL	11730	
PROLONGED/30-74MIN	99354			PNEUMONIA, >2 Y	90732		NAIL REMOVAL, W/ MATRIX	11750	
SPECIAL REPORTS/FORMS	99080			PNEUMONIA CONJUGATE, <5Y	90669		SKIN TA, 1-15	11200	
DISABILITY/WORKERS COMP	99455			TD, > 7Y	90718		DENTAL (For practice purposes only)		
SPECIMIN HANDLING	99000			VARICELLA	90716		PERIODIC ORAL EVALUATION	DE0100	
OFFICE PROCEDURES				LABORATORY			COMPREHENSIVE EVALUATION	(DE0150)	150.00
ANOSCOPY	46600			VENIPUNCTURE	36415		INTRAORAL, PERIAPICAL – 1ST FILM	(DE0200)	25.00
AUDIOMETRY	92551			BLOOD GLUCOSE, MONITORING DEVICE	82962		INTRAORAL, PERIAPICAL–EACH ADD'L FILM	(DE0250)	30.00 x2
CERUMEN REMOVAL	69210			BLOOD GLUCOSE, VISUAL DIPSTICK	82948		BITEWING	(DE026-)	42.00
COLPOSCOPY	54752			CBC, W/ AUTO DIFFERENTIAL	85025		PROPHYLAXIS - ADULT	(DE1000)	64.00
COLPOSCOPY W/ BIOPSY	57455			CBC, W/O AUTO DIFFRENTIAL	85027		PROPHYLAXIS - CHILD	DE2000	
ECG W/ INTERPRETATION	93000			CHOLESTEROL	82465		PERIODONTAL MAINT.	DE5000	
ECG, RHYTHM STRIP	93040			HEMOOCULT, GUAIAC	82272		RESTORATIVE (ANTERIOR)	DE250-	
ENDOMETRIAL BIOPSY	58100			HEMOCCULT, IMMUNOASSAY	82274		RESTORATIVE (POSTERIOR)	DE260-	
FLEXIBLE SIGMOIDOSCOPY	45330			HEMOGLOBIN A1C	83036		FUSE CROWN-PORC	DE2700	
FLEXIBLE SIGMOIDOSCOPY W/ BIOPSY	45331			LIPID PANEL	80061		RE-CEMENT CROWN	DE2900	
FRACTURE CARE, CAST/SPLINT	29---			LIVER PANEL	80076		CORE BUILD UP INC. PINS	DE3000	
NEBULIZER	94640			KHO PREP (SKIN, HAIR, NAILS)	87220		CORE BUILD UP, PREFAB POST	DE3250	
NEBULIZER DEMO	94664			METABOLIC PANEL, BASIC	80048		LABIAL VENEER	DE3500	
SPIROMETRY	94010			METABOLIC PANEL, COMPHREHENSIVE	80053		CROWN - PORCELAIN FUSED TO GOLD	DE6000	
SPIROMETRY, PRE AND POST	94060			MONONUCLEOSIS	86663		CROWN LENGTHENING	DE4000	
TYMPANOMETRY	92567			PREGNANCY, BLOOD	84702		SURGICAL EXTRACTION	DE7000	
VASECTOMY	55250			PREGNANCY, URINE	81025		IMPACTED EXTRACTION	DE7250	
MEDICATIONS				RENAL PANEL	80069		LTD. ORTHO TREATMENT, ADULT	DE8000	
AMPICILIN, UP TO 500MG	J0290			SEDIMENTATION RATE	85652		ANALGESIA, NITROUS OXIDE	DE9000	

TODAY'S FEE		341.00
AMOUNT RECEIVED		0.00
BALANCE		341.00

WALDEN-MARTIN
FAMILY MEDICAL CLINIC
1234 ANYSTREET | ANYTOWN, ANYSTATE 12345
PHONE 123-123-1234 | FAX 123-123-5678

JULIE WALDEN MD
JAMES MARTIN MD
DAVID KAHN MD
ANGELA PEREZ MD
PATRICK TAYLOR DDS
JEAN BURKE NP

PATIENT INFO

First Name	MI	Last Name	Date of Birth	Sex
Marcie		Anderson	5/8/83	F

SSN	Preferred Phone	Dental Insurance	Responsible Party
651-58-1705	123-865-0987	None/Self-pay	Self

BRIEF HISTORY

Last Visit	Treatment	X-Rays: Y / N
N/A	—	

CLINICAL DATA

General Condition of Teeth
Light plague, Light Stains

General Condition of Gums
Normal

General Condition of the Floor of the Mouth
Normal

Examination and treatment plan—List in order from tooth no. 1 through no. 32—Use charting system shown

Identify missing teeth with "x"	Tooth # or letter	Surface	Description of service (including x-ray, prophylaxis, materials used, etc.)	Date service performed Mo./Day/Year	Procedure number
Upper / Right / Primary / Permanent / Left / Lower					

Remarks for unusual services

Follow up:
6 Months

Case #2

Cecil Whitver calls the office wanting to see Dr. Kahn today to look at a lump on his neck that his wife is worried might be cancer. He told his wife weeks ago that he would schedule this appointment but forgot and would like to see the doctor as soon as possible. You see that Dr. Kahn has an opening later this morning at 10:00 AM. Use the information on Mr. Whitver's patient information form and insurance card (Figure 6-3) to register him and schedule a 30-minute New Patient Visit with Dr. Kahn this morning beginning at 10:00 AM.

After Mr. Whitver is seen, Dr. Kahn asks you to start the encounter using the Chief Complaint of "Localized swelling, mass and lump, neck." Use the instructions below to complete this:

1. Click the Find Patient button at the top of the screen.
2. Enter Whitver into the Last Name search field and select the Go button.
3. If Cecil Whitver was registered correctly, his name should populate in the search results. Select the radio button next to it and click Select.
4. Select Office Visit from the left Info Panel.
5. Select today's date from the calendar picker.
6. Select New Patient from the Visit Type dropdown menu and click the Save button.
7. Select Chief Complaint from the Record dropdown menu.
8. Enter "Localized swelling, mass and lump, neck" in the Chief Complaint Box.
9. Scroll down and enter "David Kahn" in the Entry By field.
10. Click the Save Button.

At the end of the day, Mr. Whitver's encounter is coded and you are provided with the following paper encounter form to complete the superbill and submit the claim within SimChart for the Medical Office. Make sure to post his charges to the day sheet (NOTE: He does not have a copay, and therefore did not make any payments at the time of his visit).

WALDEN-MARTIN
FAMILY MEDICAL CLINIC
1234 ANYSTREET | ANYTOWN, ANYSTATE 12345
PHONE 123-123-1234 | FAX 123-123-5678

JULIE WALDEN MD
JAMES MARTIN MD
DAVID KAHN MD
ANGELA PEREZ MD
PATRICK TAYLOR DDS
JEAN BURKE NP

PATIENT INFORMATION

First Name	MI	Last Name	Date of Birth	Sex
Cecil	P	Whitver	3/21/1938	M

SSN	Home Phone	Work Phone	Cell
709-27-1204	123-123-4567		

Home Address	City	State	Zip
123 Smith Avenue	Anytown	AL	12345-1234

Marital Status	Employer	Driver's License #
Widowed	Retired	DK97196802

Emergency Contact	Relationship to Patient	Phone Number
Barb Honaker		678-123-8910

RESPONSIBLE PARTY INFORMATION   SELF ☑

First Name	MI	Last Name	Date of Birth	Sex
Cecil	P	Whitver	3/21/1938	M

SSN	Home Phone	Work Phone	Cell
709-27-1204	123-123-4567		

Home Address	City	State	Zip
123 Smith Avenue	Anytown	AL	12345-1234

Employer		Relationship to Patient
Retired		Self

INSURANCE INFORMATION

Primary Insurance Carrier	Phone Number
Medicare	1-800-123-3333

Address	City	State	Zip
1234 Insurance Road	Anytown	AL	12345-1234

Policy Holder Name (if different from patient)	Phone	Date of Birth	Sex

Policy Number	Group Number
439136804A	

Secondary Insurance Carrier	Phone Number

Address	City	State	Zip

Policy Holder Name (if different from patient)	Phone	Date of Birth	Sex

Policy Number	Group Number

I hereby give lifetime authorization for payment of insurance benefits to be made directly to Walden-Martin Medical Group, and any assisting physicians, for services rendered. I understand that I am financially responsible for all charges whether or not they are covered by insurance. In the event of default, I agree to pay all costs of collection, and reasonable attorney's fees. I hereby authorize this healthcare provider to release all information necessary to secure the payment of benefits. I further agree that a photocopy of this agreement shall be as valid as the original.

Signature *Cecil Whitver*	Date

MEDICARE   1234 Insurance Road

MEMBER NAME: Whitver, Cecil

POLICY #: 439136804A
EFFECTIVE DATE: 3/20/2015

Is entitled to:
HOSPITAL   (PART A)
MEDICAL   (PART B)

CLAIMS/INQUIRIES: 1-800-123-3333

Figure 6-3 Patient Information Form and Insurance Card for Cecil Whitver.

WALDEN-MARTIN
FAMILY MEDICAL CLINIC
1234 ANYSTREET | ANYTOWN, ANYSTATE 12345
PHONE 123-123-1234 | FAX 123-123-5678

JULIE WALDEN MD
JAMES MARTIN MD
DAVID KAHN MD
ANGELA PEREZ MD
PATRICK TAYLOR DDS
JEAN BURKE NP

Patient Name: Whitver, Cecil
DOS: [TODAY]
Diagnoses 1): R22.1
2):
3):
4):

SERVICE	CODE New	Est.	PRICE	SERVICE	CODE	PRICE	SERVICE	CODE	PRICE
OFFICE VISIT	New	Est.		MEDICATIONS CONT'D			LABORATORY CONT'D		
MINIMAL OFFICE VISIT (OV)	99201	99211		B-12, UP TO 1,000MCG	J3420		STREP, RAPID	87880	
PROBLEM FOCUSED OV	99202	99212	50.00	EPINEPHINE, UP TO 1ML	J0170		STREP CULTURE	87081	
EXPANDED OV	99203	99213		KENALOG, 10MG	J3301		TB	87116	
DETAILED OV	99204	99214		LIDCAINE, 10MG	J2001		UA, COMPLETE, NON-AUTOMATED, MICRO	81000	
COMPHREHENSIVE OV	99205	99215		PROGESTERONE, 150MG	J1055		UA, W/O MICRO NON-AUTOMATED	81002	
WELLNESS VISIT	New	Est.		RECEPHIN, 250MG	J0696		UA, W/ MICRO, NON-AUTOMATED	81001	
WELL VISIT < 1 Y	99381	99391		TESTOSTERONE, 200MG	J1080		URINE COLONY COUNT	87086	
WELL VISIT 1-4 Y	99382	99392		TIGAN, UP TO 200MG	J3250		WET MOUNT/KOH	87210	
WELL VISIT 5-11 Y	99383	99393		TORADOL, 15MG	J1885		INPATIENT/OUTPATIENT PROCEDURES		
WELL VISIT 12-17 Y	99384	99394		NORMAL SALINE, 1000CC	J7030		UPPER GI ENDOSCOPY	43235	
WELL VISIT 18-39 Y	99385	99395		PHENERGAN, UP TO 50MG	J2550		UPPER GI ENDOSCOPY W/ BIOPSY	43239	
WELL VISIT 40-64 Y	99386	99396		IMMUNIZATIONS & INJECTIONS			UPPER GI ENDOSCOPY W/ GUIDE WIRE	43248	
WELL VISIT 65 Y+	99387	99397		ALLERGEN, ONE	95115		UPPER GI ENDOSCOPY W/ BALLOON	43249	
PREVENTATIVE SERVICES				ALLERGEN, MULTIPLE	95117		COLONOSCOPY	45378	
PAP	Q0091			IMM ADMIN, ONE	90471		COLONOSCOPY W/ BIOPSY	45380	
PELVIC & BREAST	G0101			IMM ADMIN, EACH ADD'L	90472		COLONOSCOPY W/ BIOPSY REMOVAL	45384	
PROSTATE/PSA	G0103			IMM ADMIN, INTRANASAL, ONE	90473		COLONOSCOPY W/ SNARE REMOVAL	45385	
TOBACCO COUNSELING/3-10MIN	99406			IMM ADMIN, INTRANASAL, EACH ADD'L	90475		SKIN PROCEDURES		
TOBACCO COUNSELING/>10MIN	99407			INJECTION, JOINT, SMALL	206--		BURN CARE, INITIAL	16000	
WELCOME TO MEDICARE EXAM	G0366			INJECTION, THER/PROPH/DIAG	90772		FROEIGN BODY, SKIN, SIMPLE	10120	
ECG W/ WELCOME TO MEDICARE EXAM	G0366			INJECTION, TRIGGER POINT	20552		FOREIGN BODY, SKIN, COMPLEX	12121	
FLEXIBLE SIGMOIDOSCOPY	G0104			VACCINES			I&D, ABSCESS	10060	
HEMOCCULT, GUAIAC	G0107			DT, <7 Y	90702		I&D, HEMATOMA/SEROMA	10140	
FLU ADMINISTRATION	G0008			DTP	90701		LCERATION REPAIR, SIMPLE	120--	
PENUMONIA ADMINISTRATION	G0009			DTAP, <7 Y	90700		LACERATION REPAIR, LAYERED	120--	
CONSULTATION/PRE-OP CLEARANCE				FLU, 6-35 MONTHS	90657		LESION, BIOPSY, ONE	11100	69.58
EXPANDED PROBLEM FOCUSED	99242			FLU, 3Y+	90658		LESION, BIOPSY, EACH ADD'L	11101	
DETAILED	99243			HEP A, PED/ADOL, 2 DOSE	90633		LESION, DEST., BENIGN 1-14	17110	
COMPREHENSIVE/MOD COMPLEXITY	99244			HEP A, ADULT	90632		LESION DEST., PRE-MAL., SINGLE	17000	
COMPREHENSIVE/HIGH COMPLEXITY	99245			HEP B, PED/ADOL, 3 DOSE	90744		LESION DEST., PRE-MAL., EACH ADD'L	17003	
OTHER SERVICES				HEP B, ADULT	90746		LESION, EXCISION BENIGN	114--	
AFTER POSTED HOURS	99050			HEP B-HIB	90748		LESION, EXCISION, MALIGNANT	116--	
EVENING/WEEKEND APPT.	99051			HIB, 4 DOSE	90645		LESION, PARING/CUTTING, ONE	11055	
HOME HEALTH CERTIFICATION	G0180			HPV	90649		LESION PARING/CUTTING 2-4	11056	
HOME HEALTH RECERTIFICATION	G0179			IPV	90713		LESION, SHAVE	113--	
POST-OP FOLLOW UP	99024			MMR	90707		NAIL REMOVAL, PARTIAL	11730	
PROLONGED/30-74MIN	99354			PNEUMONIA, >2 Y	90732		NAIL REMOVAL, W/ MATRIX	11750	
SPECIAL REPORTS/FORMS	99080			PNEUMONIA CONJUGATE, <5Y	90669		SKIN TA, 1-15	11200	
DISABILITY/WORKERS COMP	99455			TD, > 7Y	90718		DENTAL (For practice purposes only)		
SPECIMIN HANDLING	99000			VARICELLA	90716		PERIODIC ORAL EVALUATION	DE0100	
OFFICE PROCEDURES				LABORATORY			COMPREHENSIVE EVALUATION	DE0150	
ANOSCOPY	46600			VENIPUNCTURE	36415		INTRAORAL, PERIAPICAL – 1ST FILM	DE0200	
AUDIOMETRY	92551			BLOOD GLUCOSE, MONITORING DEVICE	82962		INTRAORAL, PERIAPICAL–EACH ADD'L FILM	DE0250	
CERUMEN REMOVAL	69210			BLOOD GLUCOSE, VISUAL DIPSTICK	82948		BITEWING	DE026-	
COLPOSCOPY	54752			CBC, W/ AUTO DIFFERENTIAL	85025		PROPHYLAXIS - ADULT	DE1000	
COLPOSCOPY W/ BIOPSY	57455			CBC, W/O AUTO DIFFRENTIAL	85027		PROPHYLAXIS - CHILD	DE2000	
ECG W/ INTERPRETATION	93000			CHOLESTEROL	82465		PERIODONTAL MAINT.	DE5000	
ECG, RHYTHM STRIP	93040			HEMOOCULT, GUAIAC	82272		RESTORATIVE (ANTERIOR)	DE250-	
ENDOMETRIAL BIOPSY	58100			HEMOCCULT, IMMUNOASSAY	82274		RESTORATIVE (POSTERIOR)	DE260-	
FLEXIBLE SIGMOIDOSCOPY	45330			HEMOGLOBIN A1C	83036		FUSE CROWN-PORC	DE2700	
FLEXIBLE SIGMOIDOSCOPY W/ BIOPSY	45331			LIPID PANEL	80061		RE-CEMENT CROWN	DE2900	
FRACTURE CARE, CAST/SPLINT	29---			LIVER PANEL	80076		CORE BUILD UP INC. PINS	DE3000	
NEBULIZER	94640			KHO PREP (SKIN, HAIR, NAILS)	87220		CORE BUILD UP, PREFAB POST	DE3250	
NEBULIZER DEMO	94664			METABOLIC PANEL, BASIC	80048		LABIAL VENEER	DE3500	
SPIROMETRY	94010			METABOLIC PANEL, COMPHREHENSIVE	80053		CROWN - PORCELAIN FUSED TO GOLD	DE6000	
SPIROMETRY, PRE AND POST	94060			MONONUCLEOSIS	86663		CROWN LENGTHENING	DE4000	
TYMPANOMETRY	92567			PREGNANCY, BLOOD	84702		SURGICAL EXTRACTION	DE7000	
VASECTOMY	55250			PREGNANCY, URINE	81025		IMPACTED EXTRACTION	DE7250	
MEDICATIONS				RENAL PANEL	80069		LTD. ORTHO TREATMENT, ADULT	DE8000	
AMPICILIN, UP TO 500MG	J0290			SEDIMENTATION RATE	85652		ANALGESIA, NITROUS OXIDE	DE9000	

TODAY'S FEE		119.58
AMOUNT RECEIVED		0.00
BALANCE		119.58

Case #3

Maurice Arviso calls to see if Dr. Perez has any available appointments as early as possible. He is having severe abdominal pain and says he can leave work at any time. You see that Dr. Perez has a 45-minute opening at 1:00 PM and Mr. Arviso says he will take it. Use the information on Mr. Arviso's patient information form and insurance card (Figure 6-4) to register him and schedule a 45-minute New Patient Visit with Dr. Perez this afternoon beginning at 1:00 PM.

When Mr. Arviso arrives, he provides paperwork for Dr. Perez to complete that will allow him to return to work on the following business day. You inform him that there is a $15.00 fee for the completion of this form and he writes a check to Walden-Martin Family Medical Clinic.

Dr. Perez asks you to schedule a 30-minute follow up appointment for Mr. Arviso next Wednesday at 1:00 PM. Dr. Perez has also asked you to start the encounter for her using the Chief Complaint of "General abdominal pain." Use the following instructions:

1. Click the Find Patient button at the top of the screen.
2. Enter Arviso into the Last Name search field and select the Go button.
3. If Maurice Arviso was registered correctly, his name should populate in the search results. Select the radio button next to it and click Select.
4. Select Office Visit from the left Info Panel.
5. Select today's date from the calendar picker.
6. Select New Patient Visit from the Visit Type dropdown menu and click the Save button.
7. Select Chief Complaint from the Record dropdown menu.
8. Enter "General Abdominal pain" in the Chief Complaint Box.
9. Scroll down and enter "Angela Perez" in the Entry By field.
10. Click the Save Button.

At the end of the day, Mr. Arviso's encounter is coded and you are provided with the following paper encounter form to complete the superbill and submit the claim within SimChart for the Medical Office. Make sure to post the charges and payment to the day sheet, and post the patient payment in Maurice Arviso's ledger.

 HELPFUL HINT

As mentioned earlier in the text, charges for form completion and other administrative tasks (e.g., CPT code 99080) are typically not submitted to insurance carriers. This information should be logged on Maurice Arviso's patient ledger, and eventually the Day Sheet, but do not include it on the claim submitted to his insurance company.

WALDEN-MARTIN
FAMILY MEDICAL CLINIC
1234 ANYSTREET | ANYTOWN, ANYSTATE 12345
PHONE 123-123-1234 | FAX 123-123-5678

JULIE WALDEN MD
JAMES MARTIN MD
DAVID KAHN MD
ANGELA PEREZ MD
PATRICK TAYLOR DDS
JEAN BURKE NP

PATIENT INFORMATION

First Name	MI	Last Name	Date of Birth	Sex
Maurice	P	Arviso	4/8/1955	M

SSN	Home Phone	Work Phone	Cell
440-92-1463	123-417-8744		

Home Address	City	State	Zip
1230 E. Logan Street	Anytown	AL	12345-1234

Marital Status	Employer	Driver's License #
Widowed	Anytown University	PS32625946

Emergency Contact	Relationship to Patient	Phone Number
Jonathan Arviso		123-456-9201

RESPONSIBLE PARTY INFORMATION　　　SELF ☑

First Name	MI	Last Name	Date of Birth	Sex
Maurice	P	Arviso	4/8/1955	M

SSN	Home Phone	Work Phone	Cell
440-92-1463	123-417-8744		

Home Address	City	State	Zip
1230 E. Logan Street	Anytown	AL	12345-1234

Employer	Relationship to Patient
Anytown University	Self

INSURANCE INFORMATION

Primary Insurance Carrier	Phone Number
Eagle Health	1-800-123-6666

Address	City	State	Zip
1234 Insurance Street	Anytown	AL	12345-1234

Policy Holder Name (if different from patient)	Phone	Date of Birth	Sex

Policy Number	Group Number
RT3502026	29627F

Secondary Insurance Carrier	Phone Number

Address	City	State	Zip

Policy Holder Name (if different from patient)	Phone	Date of Birth	Sex

Policy Number	Group Number

I hereby give lifetime authorization for payment of insurance benefits to be made directly to Walden-Martin Medical Group, and any assisting physicians, for services rendered. I understand that I am financially responsible for all charges whether or not they are covered by insurance. In the event of default, I agree to pay all costs of collection, and reasonable attorney's fees. I hereby authorize this healthcare provider to release all information necessary to secure the payment of benefits. I further agree that a photocopy of this agreement shall be as valid as the original.

Signature	Date
Maurice P. Arviso	

Eagle Health

MEMBER NAME: Arviso, Maurice
POLICY NUMBER: RT3502026
GROUP #: 29627F
DEPENDENTS:　　　　　　　　**EFFECTIVE DATE:** 07/27/2015

Network Coinsurance:　　　　Care RX:
In: 90% / 10%　　　　　　Rx Bin:　840513
Out: 70% / 30%　　　　　Rx Group: 6410RX

CLAIMS/INQUIRIES: 1-800-123-6666

Figure 6-4 Patient Information Form and Insurance Card for Maurice Arviso.

WALDEN-MARTIN
FAMILY MEDICAL CLINIC
1234 ANYSTREET | ANYTOWN, ANYSTATE 12345
PHONE 123-123-1234 | FAX 123-123-5678

JULIE WALDEN MD
JAMES MARTIN MD
DAVID KAHN MD
(ANGELA PEREZ MD)
PATRICK TAYLOR DDS
JEAN BURKE NP

Patient Name: Arviso, Maurice
DOS: [TODAY]
Diagnoses 1): R10.84
2):
3):
4):

SERVICE	CODE New	CODE Est.	PRICE
OFFICE VISIT	New	Est.	
MINIMAL OFFICE VISIT (OV)	99201	99211	
PROBLEM FOCUSED OV	(99202)	99212	50.00
EXPANDED OV	99203	99213	
DETAILED OV	99204	99214	
COMPHREHENSIVE OV	99205	99215	
WELLNESS VISIT	New	Est.	
WELL VISIT < 1 Y	99381	99391	
WELL VISIT 1-4 Y	99382	99392	
WELL VISIT 5-11 Y	99383	99393	
WELL VISIT 12-17 Y	99384	99394	
WELL VISIT 18-39 Y	99385	99395	
WELL VISIT 40-64 Y	99386	99396	
WELL VISIT 65 Y+	99387	99397	
PREVENTATIVE SERVICES			
PAP	Q0091		
PELVIC & BREAST	G0101		
PROSTATE/PSA	G0103		
TOBACCO COUNSELING/3-10MIN	99406		
TOBACCO COUNSELING/>10MIN	99407		
WELCOME TO MEDICARE EXAM	G0366		
ECG W/ WELCOME TO MEDICARE EXAM	G0366		
FLEXIBLE SIGMOIDOSCOPY	G0104		
HEMOCCULT, GUAIAC	G0107		
FLU ADMINISTRATION	G0008		
PENUMONIA ADMINISTRATION	G0009		
CONSULTATION/PRE-OP CLEARANCE			
EXPANDED PROBLEM FOCUSED	99242		
DETAILED	99243		
COMPREHENSIVE/MOD COMPLEXITY	99244		
COMPREHENSIVE/HIGH COMPLEXITY	99245		
OTHER SERVICES			
AFTER POSTED HOURS	99050		
EVENING/WEEKEND APPT.	99051		
HOME HEALTH CERTIFICATION	G0180		
HOME HEALTH RECERTIFICATION	G0179		
POST-OP FOLLOW UP	99024		
PROLONGED/30-74MIN	99354		
SPECIAL REPORTS/FORMS	(99080)		15.00
DISABILITY/WORKERS COMP	99455		
SPECIMIN HANDLING	99000		
OFFICE PROCEDURES			
ANOSCOPY	46600		
AUDIOMETRY	92551		
CERUMEN REMOVAL	69210		
COLPOSCOPY	54752		
COLPOSCOPY W/ BIOPSY	57455		
ECG W/ INTERPRETATION	93000		
ECG, RHYTHM STRIP	93040		
ENDOMETRIAL BIOPSY	58100		
FLEXIBLE SIGMOIDOSCOPY	45330		
FLEXIBLE SIGMOIDOSCOPY W/ BIOPSY	45331		
FRACTURE CARE, CAST/SPLINT	29---		
NEBULIZER	94640		
NEBULIZER DEMO	94664		
SPIROMETRY	94010		
SPIROMETRY, PRE AND POST	94060		
TYMPANOMETRY	92567		
VASECTOMY	55250		
MEDICATIONS			
AMPICILIN, UP TO 500MG	J0290		

SERVICE	CODE	PRICE
MEDICATIONS CONT'D		
B-12, UP TO 1,000MCG	J3420	
EPINEPHINE, UP TO 1ML	J0170	
KENALOG, 10MG	J3301	
LIDCAINE, 10MG	J2001	
PROGESTERONE, 150MG	J1055	
RECEPHIN, 250MG	J0696	
TESTOSTERONE, 200MG	J1080	
TIGAN, UP TO 200MG	J3250	
TORADOL, 15MG	J1885	
NORMAL SALINE, 1000CC	J7030	
PHENERGAN, UP TO 50MG	J2550	
IMMUNIZATIONS & INJECTIONS		
ALLERGEN, ONE	95115	
ALLERGEN, MULTIPLE	95117	
IMM ADMIN, ONE	90471	
IMM ADMIN, EACH ADD'L	90472	
IMM ADMIN, INTRANASAL, ONE	90473	
IMM ADMIN, INTRANASAL, EACH ADD'L	90475	
INJECTION, JOINT, SMALL	206--	
INJECTION, THER/PROPH/DIAG	90772	
INJECTION, TRIGGER POINT	20552	
VACCINES		
DT, <7 Y	90702	
DTP	90701	
DTAP, <7 Y	90700	
FLU, 6-35 MONTHS	90657	
FLU, 3Y+	90658	
HEP A, PED/ADOL, 2 DOSE	90633	
HEP A, ADULT	90632	
HEP B, PED/ADOL, 3 DOSE	90744	
HEP B, ADULT	90746	
HEP B-HIB	90748	
HIB, 4 DOSE	90645	
HPV	90649	
IPV	90713	
MMR	90707	
PNEUMONIA, >2 Y	90732	
PNEUMONIA CONJUGATE, <5Y	90669	
TD, > 7Y	90718	
VARICELLA	90716	
LABORATORY		
VENIPUNCTURE	36415	
BLOOD GLUCOSE, MONITORING DEVICE	82962	
BLOOD GLUCOSE, VISUAL DIPSTICK	82948	
CBC, W/ AUTO DIFFERENTIAL	(85025)	35.00
CBC, W/O AUTO DIFFRENTIAL	85027	
CHOLESTEROL	82465	
HEMOOCULT, GUAIAC	82272	
HEMOCCULT, IMMUNOASSAY	82274	
HEMOGLOBIN A1C	83036	
LIPID PANEL	80061	
LIVER PANEL	80076	
KHO PREP (SKIN, HAIR, NAILS)	87220	
METABOLIC PANEL, BASIC	80048	
METABOLIC PANEL, COMPHREHENSIVE	80053	
MONONUCLEOSIS	86663	
PREGNANCY, BLOOD	84702	
PREGNANCY, URINE	81025	
RENAL PANEL	80069	
SEDIMENTATION RATE	85652	

SERVICE	CODE	PRICE
LABORATORY CONT'D		
STREP, RAPID	87880	
STREP CULTURE	87081	
TB	87116	
UA, COMPLETE, NON-AUTOMATED, MICRO	81000	
UA, W/O MICRO NON-AUTOMATED	81002	
UA, W/ MICRO, NON-AUTOMATED	81001	
URINE COLONY COUNT	(87086)	32.00
WET MOUNT/KOH	87210	
INPATIENT/OUTPATIENT PROCEDURES		
UPPER GI ENDOSCOPY	43235	
UPPER GI ENDOSCOPY W/ BIOPSY	43239	
UPPER GI ENDOSCOPY W/ GUIDE WIRE	43248	
UPPER GI ENDOSCOPY W/ BALLOON	43249	
COLONOSCOPY	45378	
COLONOSCOPY W/ BIOPSY	45380	
COLONOSCOPY W/ BIOPSY REMOVAL	45384	
COLONOSCOPY W/ SNARE REMOVAL	45385	
SKIN PROCEDURES		
BURN CARE, INITIAL	16000	
FROEIGN BODY, SKIN, SIMPLE	10120	
FOREIGN BODY, SKIN, COMPLEX	12121	
I&D, ABSCESS	10060	
I&D, HEMATOMA/SEROMA	10140	
LCERATION REPAIR, SIMPLE	120--	
LACERATION REPAIR, LAYERED	120--	
LESION, BIOPSY, ONE	11100	
LESION, BIOPSY, EACH ADD'L	11101	
LESION, DEST., BENIGN 1-14	17110	
LESION DEST., PRE-MAL., SINGLE	17000	
LESION DEST., PRE-MAL., EACH ADD'L	17003	
LESION, EXCISION BENIGN	114--	
LESION, EXCISION, MALIGNANT	116--	
LESION, PARING/CUTTING, ONE	11055	
LESION PARING/CUTTING 2-4	11056	
LESION, SHAVE	113--	
NAIL REMOVAL, PARTIAL	11730	
NAIL REMOVAL, W/ MATRIX	11750	
SKIN TA, 1-15	11200	
DENTAL (For practice purposes only)		
PERIODIC ORAL EVALUATION	DE0100	
COMPREHENSIVE EVALUATION	DE0150	
INTRAORAL, PERIAPICAL – 1ST FILM	DE0200	
INTRAORAL, PERIAPICAL--EACH ADD'L FILM	DE0250	
BITEWING	DE026-	
PROPHYLAXIS - ADULT	DE1000	
PROPHYLAXIS - CHILD	DE2000	
PERIODONTAL MAINT.	DE5000	
RESTORATIVE (ANTERIOR)	DE250-	
RESTORATIVE (POSTERIOR)	DE260-	
FUSE CROWN-PORC	DE2700	
RE-CEMENT CROWN	DE2900	
CORE BUILD UP INC. PINS	DE3000	
CORE BUILD UP, PREFAB POST	DE3500	
LABIAL VENEER	DE3500	
CROWN - PORCELAIN FUSED TO GOLD	DE6000	
CROWN LENGTHENING	DE4000	
SURGICAL EXTRACTION	DE7000	
IMPACTED EXTRACTION	DE7250	
LTD. ORTHO TREATMENT, ADULT	DE8000	
ANALGESIA, NITROUS OXIDE	DE9000	

TODAY'S FEE	132.00
AMOUNT RECEIVED	15.00
BALANCE	117.00

Comprehensive

Case #4

Dr. Walden was called in for an emergency consult at Anytown Hospital last night. She treated Robert Dailey (DOB 07/15/2013) for pneumonia. Because Robert and his family just moved to the area, they do not have a physician and would like to register with Dr. Walden. Dr. Walden has asked you to contact Robert's mother Julie to get his information and to schedule an appointment today for 2:00 PM. Use the information on Robert's patient information form and insurance card (Figure 6-5) to register him and schedule a 45-minute new patient visit with Dr. Walden this afternoon beginning at 2:00 PM.

When they arrive, Robert's mother Julie insists on making a payment to Robert's account because she knows he has coinsurance and she is anticipating a fee for last night's consult and today's office visit. She gives you $20.00 cash to apply to the balance.

After the visit Dr. Walden has also asked you to start the encounter for Robert using the Chief Complaint of "General pneumonia." Use the following instructions:

1. Click the Find Patient button at the top of the screen.
2. Enter Dailey into the Last Name search field and select the Go button.
3. If Robert Dailey was registered correctly, his name should populate in the search results. Select the radio button next to it and click Select.
4. Select Office Visit from the left Info Panel.
5. Select today's date from the calendar picker.
6. Select New Patient Visit from the Visit Type dropdown menu and click the Save button.
7. Select Chief Complaint from the Record dropdown menu.
8. Enter "Pneumonia" in the Chief Complaint Box.
9. Scroll down and enter "Julie Walden" in the Entry By field.
10. Click the Save Button.

At the end of the day, Robert's encounter is coded and you are provided with the following paper encounter form to complete the superbill and submit the claim within SimChart for the Medical Office. Make sure to post the charges and payment to the day sheet, and post the patient payment in Robert Dailey's ledger.

WALDEN-MARTIN
FAMILY MEDICAL CLINIC
1234 ANYSTREET | ANYTOWN, ANYSTATE 12345
PHONE 123-123-1234 | FAX 123-123-5678

JULIE WALDEN MD
JAMES MARTIN MD
DAVID KAHN MD
ANGELA PEREZ MD
PATRICK TAYLOR DDS
JEAN BURKE NP

PATIENT INFORMATION

First Name	MI	Last Name		Date of Birth	Sex
Robert		Dailey		7/15/2013	M

SSN	Home Phone	Work Phone		Cell	
841-99-9911	123-863-4712				

Home Address	City		State	Zip
9500 Wilmore Dr.	Anytown		AL	12345-1234

Marital Status	Employer	Driver's License #
Single	None	

Emergency Contact	Relationship to Patient	Phone Number
Julie Dailey	Mother	123-863-4712

RESPONSIBLE PARTY INFORMATION   SELF ☐

First Name	MI	Last Name		Date of Birth	Sex
Julie		Dailey		12/20/1987	F

SSN	Home Phone	Work Phone		Cell	
570-57-2571	123-863-4712				

Home Address	City		State	Zip
9500 Wilmore Dr.	Anytown		AL	12345-1234

Employer		Relationship to Patient
Anytown Diner		Mother

INSURANCE INFORMATION

Primary Insurance Carrier	Phone Number
Health First	1-800-123-7777

Address	City		State	Zip
1234 Insurance Boulevard	Anytown		AL	12345-1234

Policy Holder Name (if different from patient)	Phone	Date of Birth	Sex
Julie Dailey	123-863-4712	12/20/1987	F

Policy Number	Group Number	
WV8453799	53806R	

Secondary Insurance Carrier	Phone Number

Address	City		State	Zip

Policy Holder Name (if different from patient)	Phone	Date of Birth	Sex

Policy Number	Group Number

I hereby give lifetime authorization for payment of insurance benefits to be made directly to Walden-Martin Medical Group, and any assisting physicians, for services rendered. I understand that I am financially responsible for all charges whether or not they are covered by insurance. In the event of default, I agree to pay all costs of collection, and reasonable attorney's fees. I hereby authorize this healthcare provider to release all information necessary to secure the payment of benefits. I further agree that a photocopy of this agreement shall be as valid as the original.

Signature *Robert Dailey*	Date

HealthFirst

MEMBER NAME: Dailey, Julie
POLICY NUMBER: WV8453799
GROUP #: 53806R
DEPENDENTS: Dailey, Robert   **EFFECTIVE DATE:** 11/24/2015

Network Coinsurance: DRUG CO-PAY
In: 80% / 20%   GENERIC: $20
Out: 60% / 40%   NAME BRAND: $50

CLAIMS/INQUIRIES: 1-800-123-7777

Figure 6-5 Patient Information Form and Insurance Card for Robert Dailey.

Comprehensive

WALDEN-MARTIN
FAMILY MEDICAL CLINIC
1234 ANYSTREET | ANYTOWN, ANYSTATE 12345
PHONE 123-123-1234 | FAX 123-123-5678

JULIE WALDEN MD
JAMES MARTIN MD
DAVID KAHN MD
ANGELA PEREZ MD
PATRICK TAYLOR DDS
JEAN BURKE NP

Patient Name: Dailey, Robert
DOS: [TODAY]
Diagnoses 1): J18.9
2):
3):
4):

SERVICE	CODE		PRICE	SERVICE	CODE	PRICE	SERVICE	CODE	PRICE
OFFICE VISIT	New	Est.		MEDICATIONS CONT'D			LABORATORY CONT'D		
MINIMAL OFFICE VISIT (OV)	99201	99211		B-12, UP TO 1,000MCG	J3420		STREP, RAPID	87880	
PROBLEM FOCUSED OV	99202	99212		EPINEPHINE, UP TO 1ML	J0170		STREP CULTURE	87081	
EXPANDED OV	99203	99213	70.00	KENALOG, 10MG	J3301		TB	87116	
DETAILED OV	99204	99214		LIDCAINE, 10MG	J2001		UA, COMPLETE, NON-AUTOMATED, MICRO	81000	
COMPHREHENSIVE OV	99205	99215		PROGESTERONE, 150MG	J1055		UA, W/O MICRO NON-AUTOMATED	81002	
WELLNESS VISIT	New	Est.		RECEPHIN, 250MG	J0696		UA, W/ MICRO, NON-AUTOMATED	81001	
WELL VISIT < 1 Y	99381	99391		TESTOSTERONE, 200MG	J1080		URINE COLONY COUNT	87086	
WELL VISIT 1-4 YH	99382	99392		TIGAN, UP TO 200MG	J3250		WET MOUNT/KOH	87210	
WELL VISIT 5-11 Y	99383	99393		TORADOL, 15MG	J1885		INPATIENT/OUTPATIENT PROCEDURES		
WELL VISIT 12-17 Y	99384	99394		NORMAL SALINE, 1000CC	J7030		UPPER GI ENDOSCOPY	43235	
WELL VISIT 18-39 Y	99385	99395		PHENERGAN, UP TO 50MG	J2550		UPPER GI ENDOSCOPY W/ BIOPSY	43239	
WELL VISIT 40-64 Y	99386	99396		IMMUNIZATIONS & INJECTIONS			UPPER GI ENDOSCOPY W/ GUIDE WIRE	43248	
WELL VISIT 65 Y+	99387	99397		ALLERGEN, ONE	95115		UPPER GI ENDOSCOPY W/ BALLOON	43249	
PREVENTATIVE SERVICES				ALLERGEN, MULTIPLE	95117		COLONOSCOPY	45378	
PAP	Q0091			IMM ADMIN, ONE	90471		COLONOSCOPY W/ BIOPSY	45380	
PELVIC & BREAST	G0101			IMM ADMIN, EACH ADD'L	90472		COLONOSCOPY W/ BIOPSY REMOVAL	45384	
PROSTATE/PSA	G0103			IMM ADMIN, INTRANASAL, ONE	90473		COLONOSCOPY W/ SNARE REMOVAL	45385	
TOBACCO COUNSELING/3-10MIN	99406			IMM ADMIN, INTRANASAL, EACH ADD'L	90475		SKIN PROCEDURES		
TOBACCO COUNSELING/>10MIN	99407			INJECTION, JOINT, SMALL	206--		BURN CARE, INITIAL	16000	
WELCOME TO MEDICARE EXAM	G0366			INJECTION, THER/PROPH/DIAG	90772		FROEIGN BODY, SKIN, SIMPLE	10120	
ECG W/ WELCOME TO MEDICARE EXAM	G0366			INJECTION, TRIGGER POINT	20552		FOREIGN BODY, SKIN, COMPLEX	12121	
FLEXIBLE SIGMOIDOSCOPY	G0104			VACCINES			I&D, ABSCESS	10060	
HEMOCCULT, GUAIAC	G0107			DT, <7 Y	90702		I&D, HEMATOMA/SEROMA	10140	
FLU ADMINISTRATION	G0008			DTP	90701		LCERATION REPAIR, SIMPLE	120--	
PENUMONIA ADMINISTRATION	G0009			DTAP, <7 Y	90700		LACERATION REPAIR, LAYERED	120--	
CONSULTATION/PRE-OP CLEARANCE				FLU, 6-35 MONTHS	90657		LESION, BIOPSY, ONE	11100	
EXPANDED PROBLEM FOCUSED	99242			FLU, 3Y+	90658		LESION, BIOPSY, EACH ADD'L	11101	
DETAILED	99243			HEP A, PED/ADOL, 2 DOSE	90633		LESION, DEST., BENIGN 1-14	17110	
COMPREHENSIVE/MOD COMPLEXITY	99244			HEP A, ADULT	90632		LESION DEST., PRE-MAL., SINGLE	17000	
COMPREHENSIVE/HIGH COMPLEXITY	99245			HEP B, PED/ADOL, 3 DOSE	90744		LESION DEST., PRE-MAL., EACH ADD'L	17003	
OTHER SERVICES				HEP B, ADULT	90746		LESION, EXCISION BENIGN	114--	
AFTER POSTED HOURS	99050			HEP B-HIB	90748		LESION, EXCISION, MALIGNANT	116--	
EVENING/WEEKEND APPT.	99051			HIB, 4 DOSE	90645		LESION, PARING/CUTTING, ONE	11055	
HOME HEALTH CERTIFICATION	G0180			HPV	90649		LESION PARING/CUTTING 2-4	11056	
HOME HEALTH RECERTIFICATION	G0179			IPV	90713		LESION, SHAVE	113--	
POST-OP FOLLOW UP	99024			MMR	90707		NAIL REMOVAL, PARTIAL	11730	
PROLONGED/30-74MIN	99354			PNEUMONIA, >2 Y	90732		NAIL REMOVAL, W/ MATRIX	11750	
SPECIAL REPORTS/FORMS	99080			PNEUMONIA CONJUGATE, <5Y	90669		SKIN TA, 1-15	11200	
DISABILITY/WORKERS COMP	99455			TD, > 7Y	90718		DENTAL (For practice purposes only)		
SPECIMIN HANDLING	99000			VARICELLA	90716		PERIODIC ORAL EVALUATION	DE0100	
OFFICE PROCEDURES				LABORATORY			COMPREHENSIVE EVALUATION	DE0150	
ANOSCOPY	46600			VENIPUNCTURE	36415		INTRAORAL, PERIAPICAL – 1ST FILM	DE0200	
AUDIOMETRY	92551			BLOOD GLUCOSE, MONITORING DEVICE	82962		INTRAORAL, PERIAPICAL–EACH ADD'L FILM	DE0250	
CERUMEN REMOVAL	69210			BLOOD GLUCOSE, VISUAL DIPSTICK	82948		BITEWING	DE026-	
COLPOSCOPY	54752			CBC, W/ AUTO DIFFERENTIAL	85025		PROPHYLAXIS - ADULT	DE1000	
COLPOSCOPY W/ BIOPSY	57455			CBC, W/O AUTO DIFFRENTIAL	85027		PROPHYLAXIS - CHILD	DE2000	
ECG W/ INTERPRETATION	93000			CHOLESTEROL	82465		PERIODONTAL MAINT.	DE5000	
ECG, RHYTHM STRIP	93040			HEMOOCULT, GUAIAC	82272		RESTORATIVE (ANTERIOR)	DE250-	
ENDOMETRIAL BIOPSY	58100			HEMOCCULT, IMMUNOASSAY	82274		RESTORATIVE (POSTERIOR)	DE260-	
FLEXIBLE SIGMOIDOSCOPY	45330			HEMOGLOBIN A1C	83036		FUSE CROWN-PORC	DE2700	
FLEXIBLE SIGMOIDOSCOPY W/ BIOPSY	45331			LIPID PANEL	80061		RE-CEMENT CROWN	DE2900	
FRACTURE CARE, CAST/SPLINT	29---			LIVER PANEL	80076		CORE BUILD UP INC. PINS	DE3000	
NEBULIZER	94640			KHO PREP (SKIN, HAIR, NAILS)	87220		CORE BUILD UP, PREFAB POST	DE3250	
NEBULIZER DEMO	94664			METABOLIC PANEL, BASIC	80048		LABIAL VENEER	DE3500	
SPIROMETRY	94010			METABOLIC PANEL, COMPHREHENSIVE	80053		CROWN - PORCELAIN FUSED TO GOLD	DE6000	
SPIROMETRY, PRE AND POST	94060			MONONUCLEOSIS	86663		CROWN LENGTHENING	DE4000	
TYMPANOMETRY	92567			PREGNANCY, BLOOD	84702		SURGICAL EXTRACTION	DE7000	
VASECTOMY	55250			PREGNANCY, URINE	81025		IMPACTED EXTRACTION	DE7250	
MEDICATIONS				RENAL PANEL	80069		LTD. ORTHO TREATMENT, ADULT	DE8000	
AMPICILIN, UP TO 500MG	J0290			SEDIMENTATION RATE	85652		ANALGESIA, NITROUS OXIDE	DE9000	

TODAY'S FEE		70.00
AMOUNT RECEIVED		20.00
BALANCE		50.00

Cumulative Paperwork

In addition to the patient visits included in the previous cases, Walden-Martin Family Medical Clinic received the following Explanation of Benefits today. Please log these payments in both the patients' ledgers and on the day sheet.

AETNA

1234 Insurance Way
Anytown, AL 12345-1234

Walden-Martin
1234 Anystreet
Anytown, AL 13245-1234

Provider: Julie Walden
Check #: 1654103
Check Date: [TODAY]
Check Amount: $110.00

DOS	Procedure	Billed	Contract Adjustment	Co-Pay	Deductible	Paid
NAME: Walter Biller				**ID#: CH8327753**		
08/28/2015	99396	$105.00	$16.00	$25.00	$14.00	$50.00
08/28/2015	85025	$35.00	$6.00	—	—	$29.00
08/28/2015	81000	$25.00	$4.00	—	—	$21.00
	CLAIM TOTALS:	$165.00	$26.00	$25.00	$14.00	$100.00
NAME: Carl Bowden				**ID#: CB5124863**		
09/01/2015	99213	$43.00	$8.00	$25.00	$0.00	$10.00
	CLAIM TOTALS:	$43.00	$8.00	$25.00	$0.00	$10.00
NAME: Erma Willis				**ID#: EW8884910**		
08/26/2015	99213	$43.00	$8.00	$25.00	$10.00	$0.00
	CLAIM TOTALS:	$43.00	$8.00	$25.00	$10.00	$0.00

MEDICARE

1234 Insurance Road
Anytown, AL 12345-1234

Provider: Jean Burke
Check #: 784137
Check Date: [TODAY]
Check Amount: $149.00

Walden-Martin
1234 Anystreet
Anytown, AL 13245-1234

DOS	Procedure	Billed	Contract Adjustment	Co-Pay	Deductible	Paid
NAME: Robert Caudill				**ID#: 312277298B**		
09/08/2015	99212	$32.00	$5.20	$25.00	—	$1.80
09/08/2015	20610	$89.00	$15.40	—	—	$73.60
09/08/2015	20610	$89.00	$15.40	—	—	$73.60
	CLAIM TOTALS:	$210.00	$36.00	$25.00	$0.00	$149.00

Comprehensive

MetLife

1234 Insurance Avenue
Anytown, AL 12345-1234

Walden-Martin
1234 Anystreet
Anytown, AL 13245-1234

Provider: Pedro Gomez
Patient ID: PG88602686
Provider: James Martin
Paid Date: [TODAY]
Check Number: 8973192

DOS	Procedure	Billed	Contract Adjustment	Co-Pay	Deductible	Paid
09/09/2015	99383	$70.00	$10.50	$25.00	$34.50	$0.00
09/09/2015	G0008	$7.00	$1.20	—	$1.50	$4.30
	TOTALS:	$77.00	$11.70	$25.00	$36.00	$4.30

Complete and save the day sheet and then complete the bank deposit slip for the evening, including Maurice Arviso's check payment (see Case #3), the cash payment for Robert Dailey's account (see Case #4), and the checks received from the insurance carriers above.

 Now complete the Review Questions for this unit on your Evolve site.

Appendix A

WALDEN-MARTIN
FAMILY MEDICAL CLINIC
1234 ANYSTREET | ANYTOWN, ANYSTATE 12345
PHONE 123-123-1234 | FAX 123-123-5678

JULIE WALDEN MD
JAMES MARTIN MD
DAVID KAHN MD
ANGELA PEREZ MD
PATRICK TAYLOR DDS
JEAN BURKE NP

Fee schedule

SERVICE	CODE	FEE
OFFICE VISIT		
NEW MINIMAL OFFICE VISIT (OV)	99201	$ 31.00
NEW PROBLEM FOCUSED OV	99202	$ 50.00
NEW EXPANDED OV	99203	$ 70.00
NEW DETAILED OV	99204	$ 89.00
NEW COMPHREHENSIVE OV	99205	$ 119.00
EST. MINIMAL OFFICE VISIT (OV)	99211	$ 24.00
EST. PROBLEM FOCUSED OV	99212	$ 32.00
EST. EXPANDED OV	99213	$ 43.00
EST. DETAILED OV	99214	$ 65.00
EST. COMPHREHENSIVE OV	99215	$ 75.00
WELLNESS VISIT		
NEW WELL VISIT < 1 Y	99381	$ 110.00
NEW WELL VISIT 1-4 Y	99382	$ 90.00
NEW WELL VISIT 5-11 Y	99383	$ 70.00
NEW WELL VISIT 12-17 Y	99384	$ 70.00
NEW WELL VISIT 18-39 Y	99385	$ 90.00
NEW WELL VISIT 40-64 Y	99386	$ 110.00
NEW WELL VISIT 65 Y+	99387	$ 135.20
EST. WELL VISIT < 1 Y	99391	$ 95.00
EST. WELL VISIT 1-4 Y	99392	$ 75.00
EST. WELL VISIT 5-11 Y	99393	$ 65.00
EST. WELL VISIT 12-17 Y	99394	$ 65.00
EST. WELL VISIT 18-39 Y	99395	$ 80.00
EST. WELL VISIT 40-64 Y	99396	$ 105.00
EST. WELL VISIT 65 Y+	99397	$ 120.00
PREVENTATIVE SERVICES		
PAP	Q0091	$ 52.00
PELVIC & BREAST	G0101	$ 79.00
PROSTATE/PSA	G0103	$ 32.10
TOBACCO COUNSELING/3-10MIN	99406	$ 17.50
TOBACCO COUNSELING/>10MIN	99407	$ 26.00
WELCOME TO MEDICARE EXAM	G0366	$ 65.50
ECG W/ WELCOME TO MEDICARE EXAM	G0366	$ 75.50
FLEXIBLE SIGMOIDOSCOPY	G0104	$ 87.60
HEMOCCULT, GUAIAC	G0107	$ 6.00
FLU ADMINISTRATION	G0008	$ 7.00
PENUMONIA ADMINISTRATION	G0009	$ 7.00
OTHER SERVICES		
AFTER POSTED HOURS	99050	$ 50.00
EVENING/WEEKEND APPT.	99051	$ 50.00
HOME HEALTH CERTIFICATION	G0180	$ 65.50
HOME HEALTH RECERTIFICATION	G0179	$ 55.00
POST-OP FOLLOW UP	99024	---
PROLONGED/30-74MIN	99354	$ 90.50
SPECIAL REPORTS/FORMS	99080	$ 15.00
DISABILITY/WORKERS COMP	99455	$ 78.00
SPECIMIN HANDLING	99000	$ 25.00

SERVICE	CODE	FEE
CONSULTATION/PRE-OP CLEARANCE		
EXPANDED PROBLEM FOCUSED	99242	$ 60.00
DETAILED	99243	$ 75.00
COMPREHENSIVE/MOD COMPLEXITY	99244	$ 90.00
COMPREHENSIVE/HIGH COMPLEXITY	99245	$ 115.00
OFFICE PROCEDURES		
ANOSCOPY	46600	$ 64.00
AUDIOMETRY	92551	$ 32.00
CERUMEN REMOVAL	69210	$ 46.00
COLPOSCOPY	54752	$ 114.00
COLPOSCOPY W/ BIOPSY	57455	$ 178.00
ECG W/ INTERPRETATION	93000	$ 89.00
ECG, RHYTHM STRIP	93040	$ 56.00
ENDOMETRIAL BIOPSY	58100	$ 152.00
FLEXIBLE SIGMOIDOSCOPY	45330	$ 90.00
FLEXIBLE SIGMOIDOSCOPY W/ BIOPSY	45331	$ 150.00
FRACTURE CARE, CAST/SPLINT	29---	$ 36.00
NEBULIZER	94640	$ 49.22
NEBULIZER DEMO	94664	$ 17.45
SPIROMETRY	94010	$ 78.00
SPIROMETRY, PRE AND POST	94060	$ 124.23
TYMPANOMETRY	92567	$ 248.57
VASECTOMY	55250	$ 345.20
MEDICATIONS		
AMPICILIN, UP TO 500MG	J0290	$ 32.00
B-12, UP TO 1,000MCG	J3420	$ 24.00
EPINEPHINE, UP TO 1ML	J0170	$ 29.79
KENALOG, 10MG	J3301	$ 34.55
LIDOCAINE, 10MG	J2001	$ 32.15
PROGESTERONE, 150MG	J1055	$ 11.50
ROCEPHIN, 250MG	J0696	$ 21.20
TESTOSTERONE, 200MG	J1080	$ 52.50
TIGAN, UP TO 200MG	J3250	$ 67.80
TORADOL, 15MG	J1885	$ 15.50
NORMAL SALINE, 1000CC	J7030	$ 17.50
PHENERGAN, UP TO 50MG	J2550	$ 21.50
IMMUNIZATIONS & INJECTIONS		
ALLERGEN, ONE	95115	$ 19.00
ALLERGEN, MULTIPLE	95117	$ 26.50
IMM ADMIN, ONE	90471	$ 10.00
IMM ADMIN, EACH ADD'L	90472	$ 10.00
IMM ADMIN, INTRANASAL, ONE	90473	$ 7.00
IMM ADMIN, INTRANASAL, EACH ADD'L	90475	$ 7.00
INJECTION, JOINT, SMALL	20600	$ 65.00
INJECTION, JOINT, INTERMEDIATE	20605	$ 75.00
INJECTION, JOINT, MAJOR	20610	$ 89.00
INJECTION, THER/PROPH/DIAG	90772	$ 25.00
INJECTION, TRIGGER POINT	20552	$ 66.00

SERVICE	CODE	FEE
VACCINES		
DT, <7 Y	90702	$ 47.50
DTP	90701	$ 49.70
DTAP, <7 Y	90700	$ 52.30
FLU, 6-35 MONTHS	90657	$ 25.50
FLU, 3Y+	90658	$ 24.00
HEP A, PED/ADOL, 2 DOSE	90633	$ 33.00
HEP A, ADULT	90632	$ 50.00
HEP B, PED/ADOL, 3 DOSE	90744	$ 78.90
HEP B, ADULT	90746	$ 66.20
HEP B-HIB	90748	$ 67.70
HIB, 4 DOSE	90645	$ 69.50
HPV	90649	$ 56.89
IPV	90713	$ 67.00
MMR	90707	$ 59.50
PNEUMONIA, >2 Y	90732	$ 45.00
PNEUMONIA CONJUGATE, <5Y	90669	$ 46.50
TD, > 7Y	90718	$ 60.00
VARICELLA	90716	$ 32.00
LABORATORY		
VENIPUNCTURE	36415	$ 10.00
BLOOD GLUCOSE, MONITORING DEVICE	82962	$ 16.00
BLOOD GLUCOSE, VISUAL DIPSTICK	82948	$ 7.00
CBC, W/ AUTO DIFFERENTIAL	85025	$ 35.00
CBC, W/O AUTO DIFFRENTIAL	85027	$ 25.00
CHOLESTEROL	82465	$ 45.00
HEMOOCULT, GUAIAC	82272	$ 7.00
HEMOCCULT, IMMUNOASSAY	82274	$ 14.00
HEMOGLOBIN A1C	83036	$ 32.00
LIPID PANEL	80061	$ 47.00
LIVER PANEL	80076	$ 39.00
KHO PREP (SKIN, HAIR, NAILS)	87220	$ 26.00
METABOLIC PANEL, BASIC	80048	$ 42.00
METABOLIC PANEL, COMPHREHENSIVE	80053	$ 55.00
MONONUCLEOSIS	86663	$ 34.00
PREGNANCY, BLOOD	84702	$ 27.00
PREGNANCY, URINE	81025	$ 18.00
RENAL PANEL	80069	$ 41.50
SEDIMENTATION RATE	85652	$ 16.00
STREP, RAPID	87880	$ 21.00
STREP CULTURE	87081	$ 38.00
TB	87116	$ 16.00
UA, COMPLETE, NON-AUTOMATED, MICRO	81000	$ 25.00
UA, W/O MICRO NON-AUTOMATED	81002	$ 22.00
UA, W/ MICRO, NON-AUTOMATED	81001	$ 27.00
URINE COLONY COUNT	87086	$ 32.00
URINE CULTURE, PRESUMPTIVE	87088	$ 39.00
WET MOUNT/KOH	87210	$ 27.00
INPATIENT/OUTPATIENT PROCEDURES		
UPPER GI ENDOSCOPY	43235	$ 136.00
UPPER GI ENDOSCOPY W/ BIOPSY	43239	$ 154.00
UPPER GI ENDOSCOPY W/ GUIDE WIRE	43248	$ 184.00
UPPER GI ENDOSCOPY W/ BALLOON	43249	$ 170.00

SERVICE	CODE	FEE
INPATIENT/OUTPATIENT PROCEDURES Contd.		
COLONOSCOPY	45378	$ 222.00
COLONOSCOPY W/ BIOPSY	45380	$ 265.00
COLONOSCOPY W/ BIOPSY REMOVAL	45384	$ 278.00
COLONOSCOPY W/ SNARE REMOVAL	45385	$ 314.00
SKIN PROCEDURES		
BURN CARE, INITIAL	16000	$ 45.00
FROEIGN BODY, SKIN, SIMPLE	10120	$ 48.00
FOREIGN BODY, SKIN, COMPLEX	12121	$ 60.00
I&D, ABSCESS	10060	$ 70.00
I&D, HEMATOMA/SEROMA	10140	$ 105.50
LCERATION REPAIR, SIMPLE	120--	$ 110.00
LACERATION REPAIR, LAYERED	120--	$ 210.45
LESION, BIOPSY, ONE	11100	$ 69.58
LESION, BIOPSY, EACH ADD'L	11101	$ 57.70
LESION, DEST., BENIGN 1-14	17110	$ 38.00
LESION DEST., PRE-MAL., SINGLE	17000	$ 26.00
LESION DEST., PRE-MAL., EACH ADD'L	17003	$ 33.20
LESION, EXCISION BENIGN	114--	$ 61.00
LESION, EXCISION, MALIGNANT	116--	$ 64.50
LESION, PARING/CUTTING, ONE	11055	$ 54.00
LESION PARING/CUTTING 2-4	11056	$ 64.00
LESION, SHAVE	113--	$ 16.00
NAIL REMOVAL, PARTIAL	11730	$ 115.00
NAIL REMOVAL, W/ MATRIX	11750	$ 164.00
SKIN TA, 1-15	11200	$ 49.00
DENTAL (For practice purposes only)		
PERIODIC ORAL EVALUATION	DE0100	$ 36.00
COMPREHENSIVE EVALUATION	DE0150	$ 150.00
INTRAORAL, PERIAPICAL – 1ST FILM	DE0200	$ 25.00
INTRAORAL, PERIAPICAL–EACH ADD'L FILM	DE0250	$ 15.00
BITEWING 1 FILM	DE0261	$ 20.00
BITEWING 2 FILMS	DE0262	$ 27.00
BITEWING 3 FILMS	DE0263	$ 42.00
PROPHYLAXIS - ADULT	DE1000	$ 64.00
PROPHYLAXIS - CHILD	DE2000	$ 50.00
PERIODONTAL MAINT.	DE5000	$ 108.00
RESTORATIVE (ANTERIOR) 1 SURFACE	DE2501	$ 117.00
RESTORATIVE (ANTERIOR) 2 SURFACES	DE2502	$ 155.00
RESTORATIVE (ANTERIOR) 3 SURFACES	DE2503	$ 186.00
RESTORATIVE (POSTERIOR) 1 SURFACE	DE2601	$ 124.00
RESTORATIVE (POSTERIOR) 2 SURFACES	DE2602	$ 189.00
RESTORATIVE (POSTERIOR) 3 SURFACES	DE2603	$ 242.00
FUSE CROWN-PORC	DE2700	$ 975.00
RE-CEMENT CROWN	DE2900	$ 82.00
CORE BUILD UP INC. PINS	DE3000	$ 210.00
CORE BUILD UP, PREFAB POST	DE3250	$ 259.00
LABIAL VENEER	DE3500	$ 847.00
CROWN - PORCELAIN FUSED TO GOLD	DE6000	$ 826.00
CROWN LENGTHENING	DE4000	$ 556.00
SURGICAL EXTRACTION	DE7000	$ 210.00
IMPACTED EXTRACTION	DE7250	$ 308.00
LTD. ORTHO TREATMENT, ADULT	DE8000	$ 2,078.00
ANALGESIA, NITROUS OXIDE	DE9000	$ 51.00